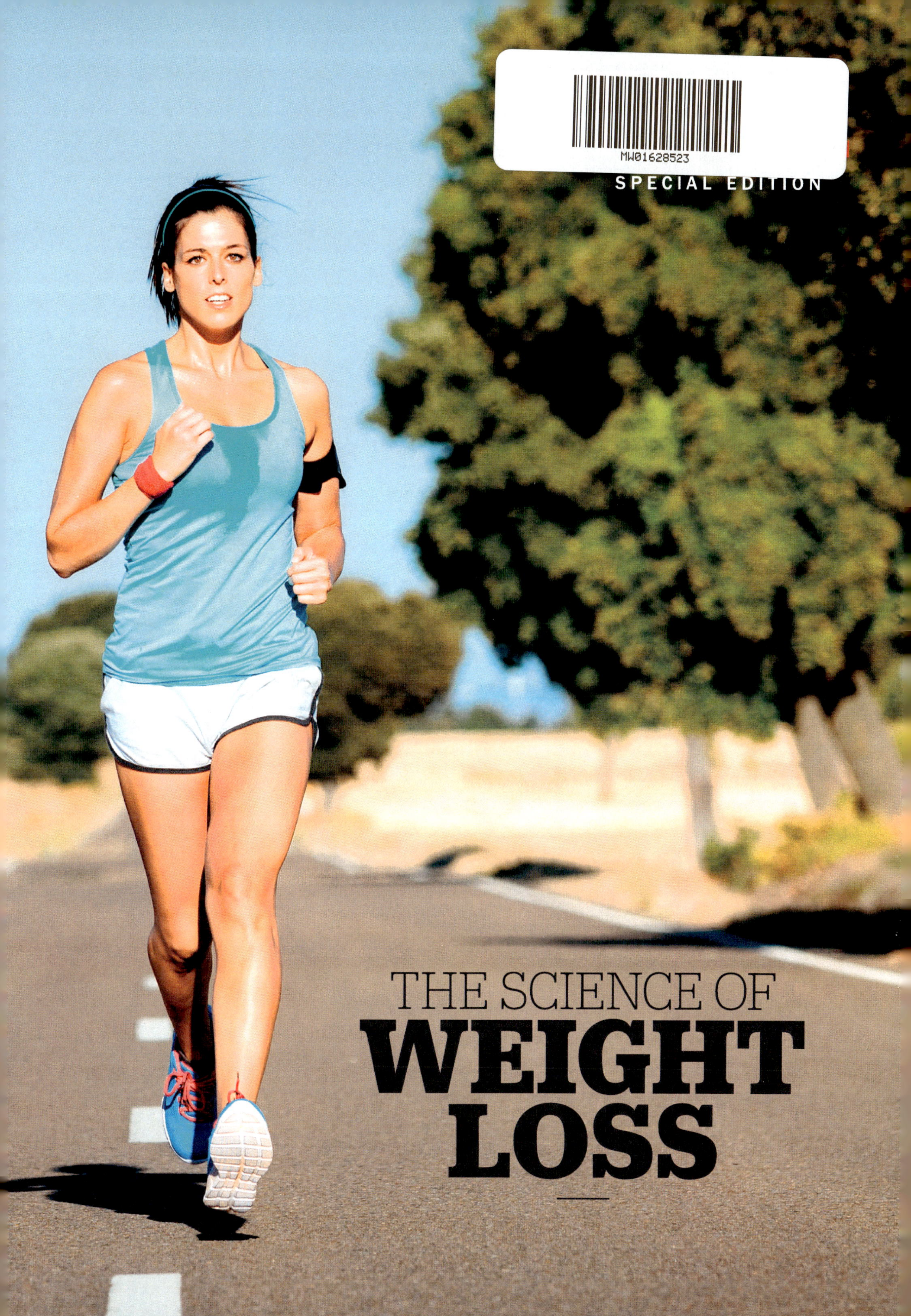

MW01628523
SPECIAL EDITION
THE SCIENCE OF
WEIGHT
LOSS

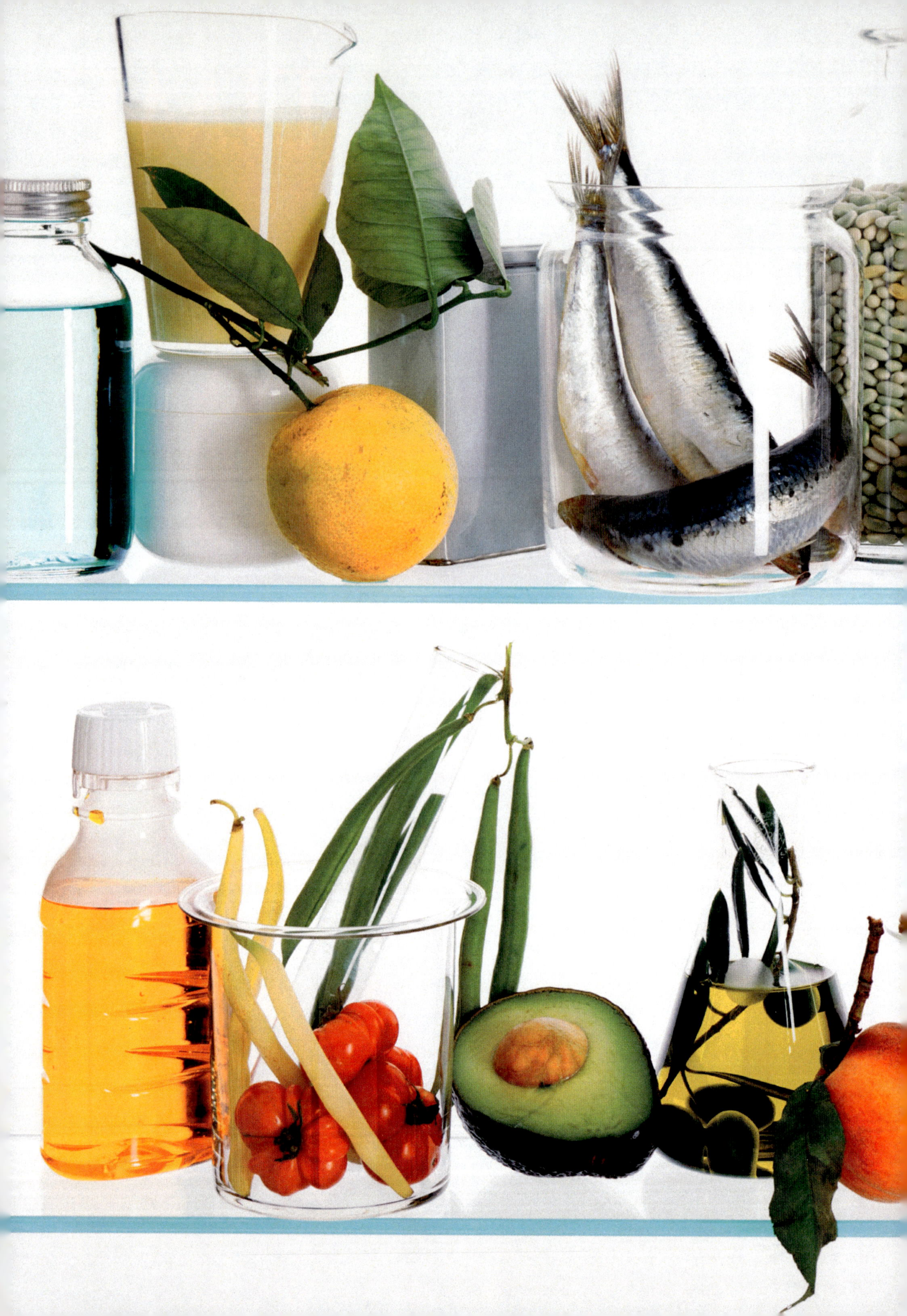

Contents

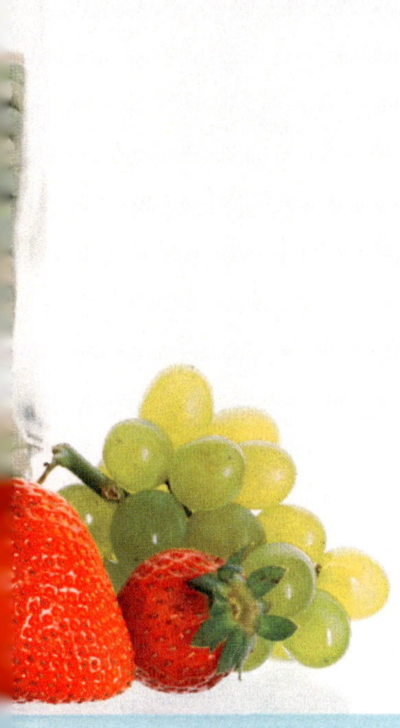

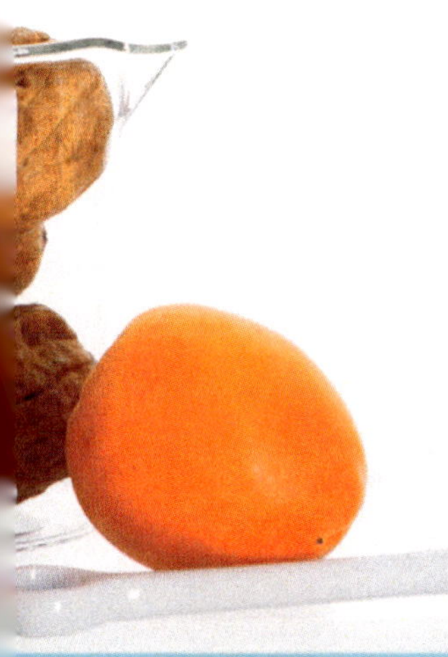

Parts of this edition appeared previously in TIME and *Health*.

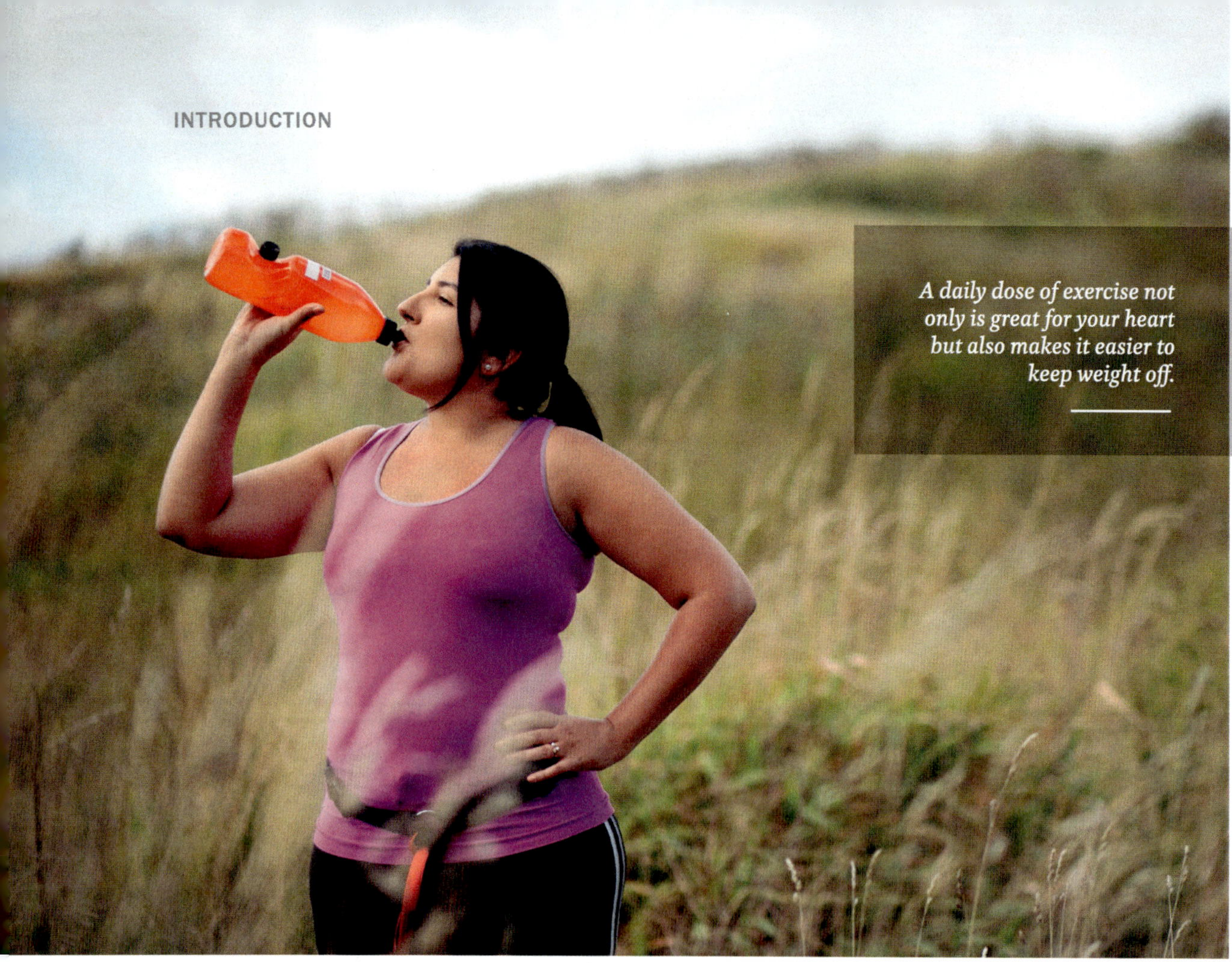

A daily dose of exercise not only is great for your heart but also makes it easier to keep weight off.

What a Healthy Diet Looks Like

The struggle to shed pounds is real. But it is possible to eat healthier and lose weight in a way that is sustainable for you

> **By Hallie Levine**

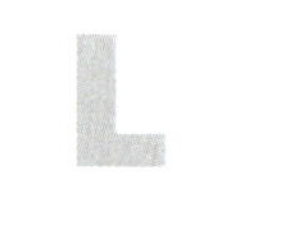

LOSING WEIGHT IS NO EASY TASK, WHICH HELPS EXPLAIN WHY THE U.S. weight-loss market is a $66 billion industry. Dropping pounds quickly or through dramatic short-term approaches is often not the best idea, yet Americans spend billions of dollars each year going on coordinated diet programs, undergoing bariatric surgery, using apps that track their every calorie and step, and even embracing "fad" diets (Paleo or keto, anyone?). And for all that, the weighty truth is that more than 70% of U.S. adults remain either overweight or obese.

On the surface, weight loss should be simple: cut back on calories, ramp up on exercise, and the pounds should fly—and stay—off. But it's much more complicated than that. "Obesity is a real disease, with real physiological consequences: when you gain weight, the nerves in your hypothalamus that conduct signals from your fat cells to the rest of your brain become damaged," explains Louis Aronne, director of the Center for Weight Management and Metabolic Clinical Research at Weill-Cornell Medical College. "As a result, your brain doesn't realize that you're full, so you keep eating."

At that point, people are not gaining weight just because they're consuming more calories—once someone has become overweight or obese, the body produces hormones such as insulin that increase fat storage. That makes it more likely that those extra noshes will be harbored as fat.

The health consequences are real. "More than 70 illnesses—including heart disease, Type 2 diabetes and even some cancers—are the direct result of carrying around too much body fat," says Aronne.

Even when people do end up shedding weight, the regain rates are staggering. More than 80% of successful dieters end up gaining back all their weight—and then some—within about two years, according to a UCLA review of more than 30 studies. Once you start losing a substantial amount of weight—considered at least 10% of your body weight—your body goes into "starvation mode." Your system slows its production of leptin, a hormone that suppresses your appetite, while at the same time pumping up levels of the hunger hormone ghrelin, explains Aronne. The result: you're walking around feeling constantly famished.

More than 80% of successful dieters end up gaining back all their weight—and then some—within about two years.

Yet despite the odds, there are encouraging signs. There is a growing movement to focus on healthy lifestyle tweaks rather than extreme diets. Recognizing this shift, in 2018 Weight Watchers rebranded itself as WW, with the slogan "Wellness That Works." Its new mission: "We inspire healthy habits for real life."

Meanwhile, researchers keep learning from people who lose pounds and get healthier as a result. "Ultimately, it doesn't matter if you put someone on a low-fat or a low-carbohydrate diet—in the end, studies show people lose the same amount of weight," says Caroline Apovian, a weight-loss specialist at the Boston University School of Medicine and the president of the Obesity Society.

Often, a lower-carbohydrate diet—one in which about 30% of calories come from protein and the rest from low-glycemic foods (those that don't raise your blood sugar quickly, such as non-starchy vegetables, nuts, beans and some fruits)—is easier to follow because it's less likely to trigger hunger pangs. "I usually encourage patients to eat as much protein, fruits and non-starchy vegetables as they want, while restricting starch intake to one to two servings a day," says Apovian. Protein is particularly essential because it helps build back muscle mass, which reverses the decline in metabolism.

When you do eat starchy carbs, try to consume them last—people who ate chicken and vegetables first, followed by bread and orange juice, had significantly lower blood-sugar and insulin levels after a meal than people who ate the exact same thing in the reverse order, according to a study by Aronne published in 2015 in the medical journal *Diabetes Care*.

Exercise is also a key piece of the puzzle. Whereas aerobic exercise helps you lose weight by increasing the amount of calories you expend, resistance training helps prevent your metabolism from taking a nosedive. That's because along with fat, you shed muscle too; and the less muscle you have, the fewer calories you burn. But a 2015 study found that healthy adults who did resistance training two to three times a week for nine months saw a 5% increase in resting metabolic rate.

Finally, don't discount the real health benefits you gain from shedding just a little bit of weight. "We see the greatest improvements in health with just losing 5% to 10% of body weight," says Aronne. Losing merely this much significantly lowered patients' risk for diabetes and cardiovascular disease, according to a 2016 study published in *Cell Metabolism*. "If someone's 200 pounds, it's a lot less daunting to encourage them to lose just 10 or 20 pounds, as opposed to 50," adds Aronne. "They're much more likely to keep off that weight."

And at the end of the day, from an overall wellness perspective, that's what matters the most. □

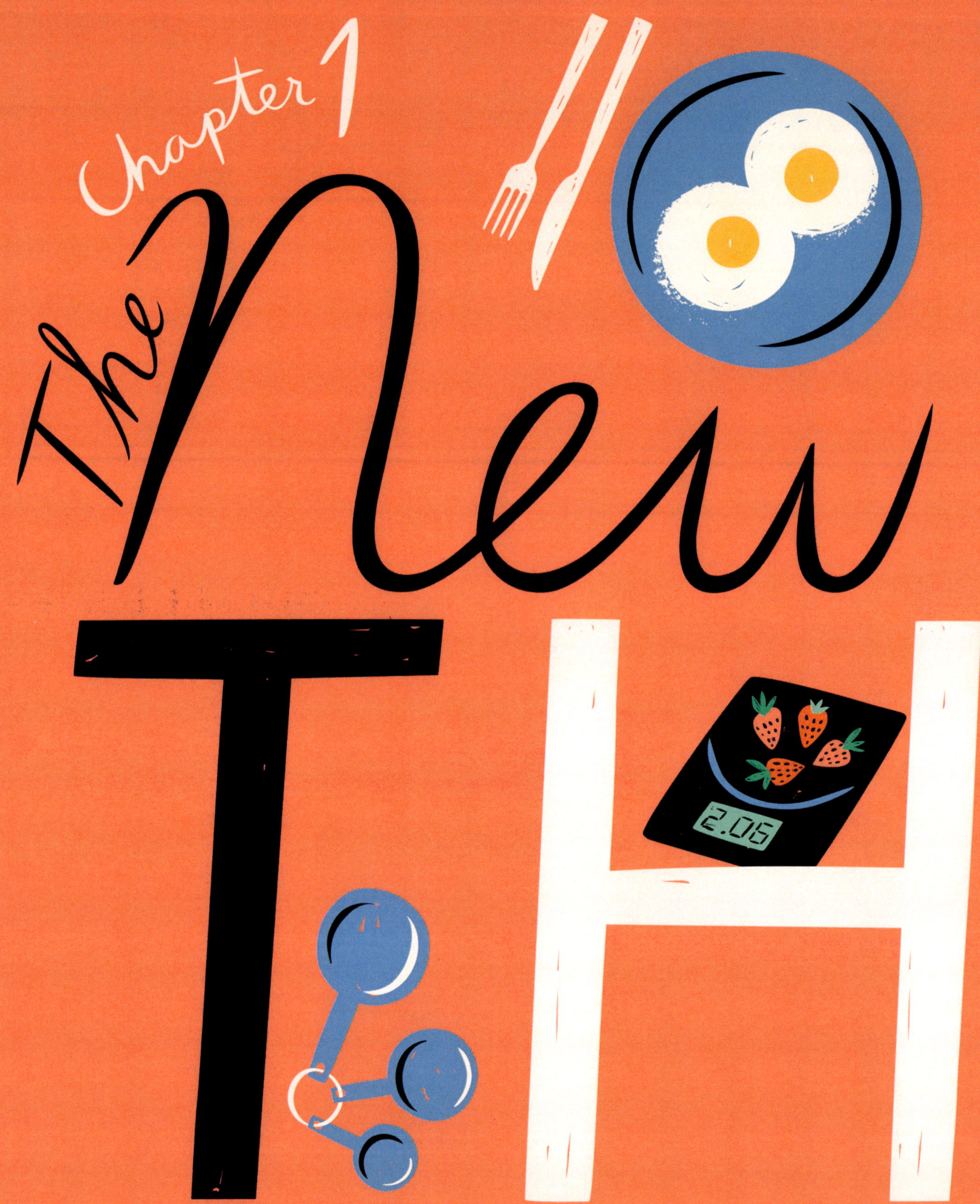

What really works, why the right calories matter,

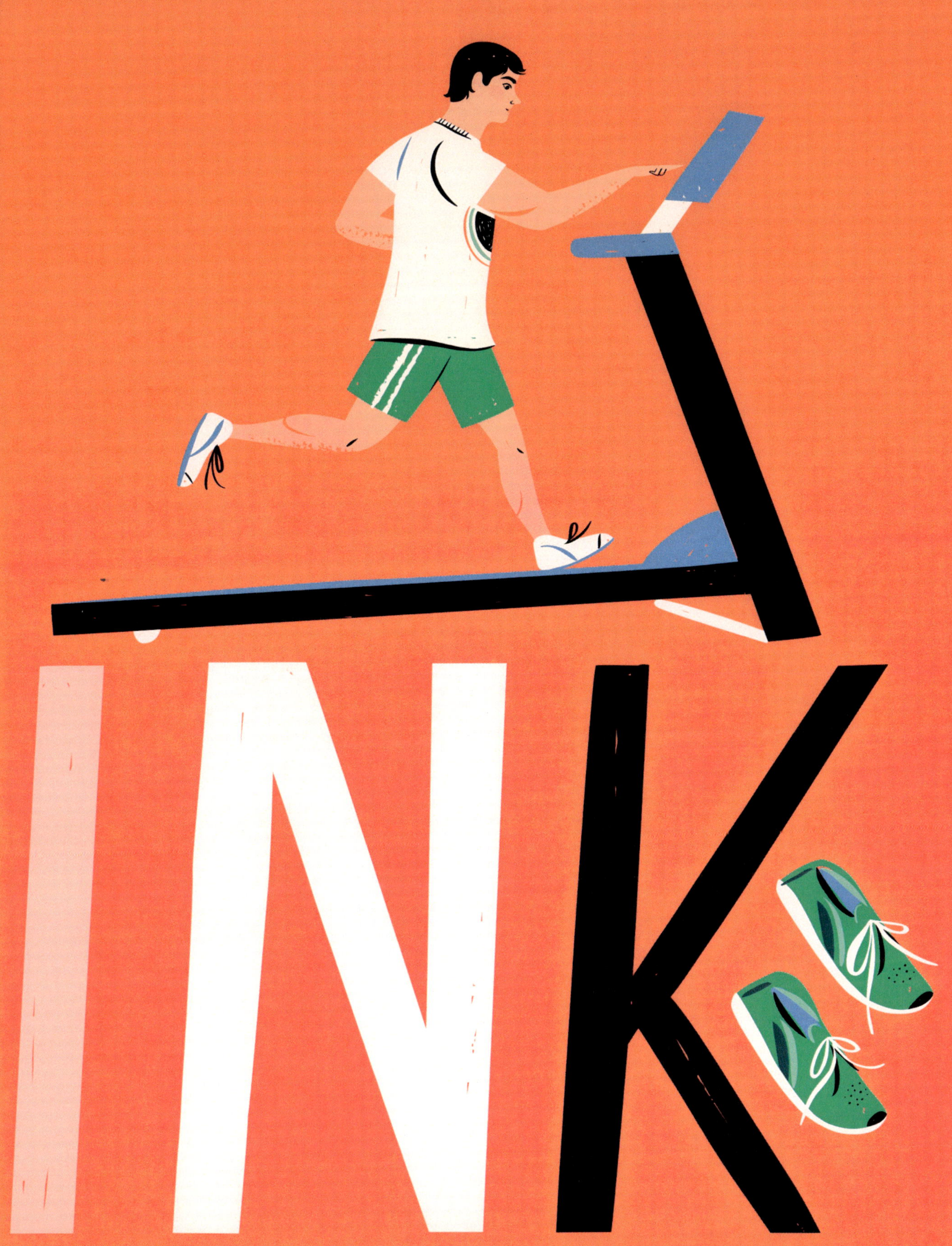

raising body-positive kids and all about body fat

Why Your Diet Isn't Working (and What to Do About It)

There is no such thing as one perfect weight-loss plan

By Alexandra Sifferlin

LIKE MOST PEOPLE, KEVIN HALL used to think the reason people get fat is simple.

"Why don't they just eat less and exercise more?" he remembers thinking. Trained as a physicist, he had always thought the calories-in-vs.-calories-burned equation for weight loss made sense. But then his own research—and the contestants on a smash reality-TV show—proved him wrong.

Hall, a scientist at the National Institutes of Health (NIH), started watching *The Biggest Loser* several years ago on the recommendation of a friend. "I saw these folks stepping on scales, and they lost 20 pounds in a week," he says. On the

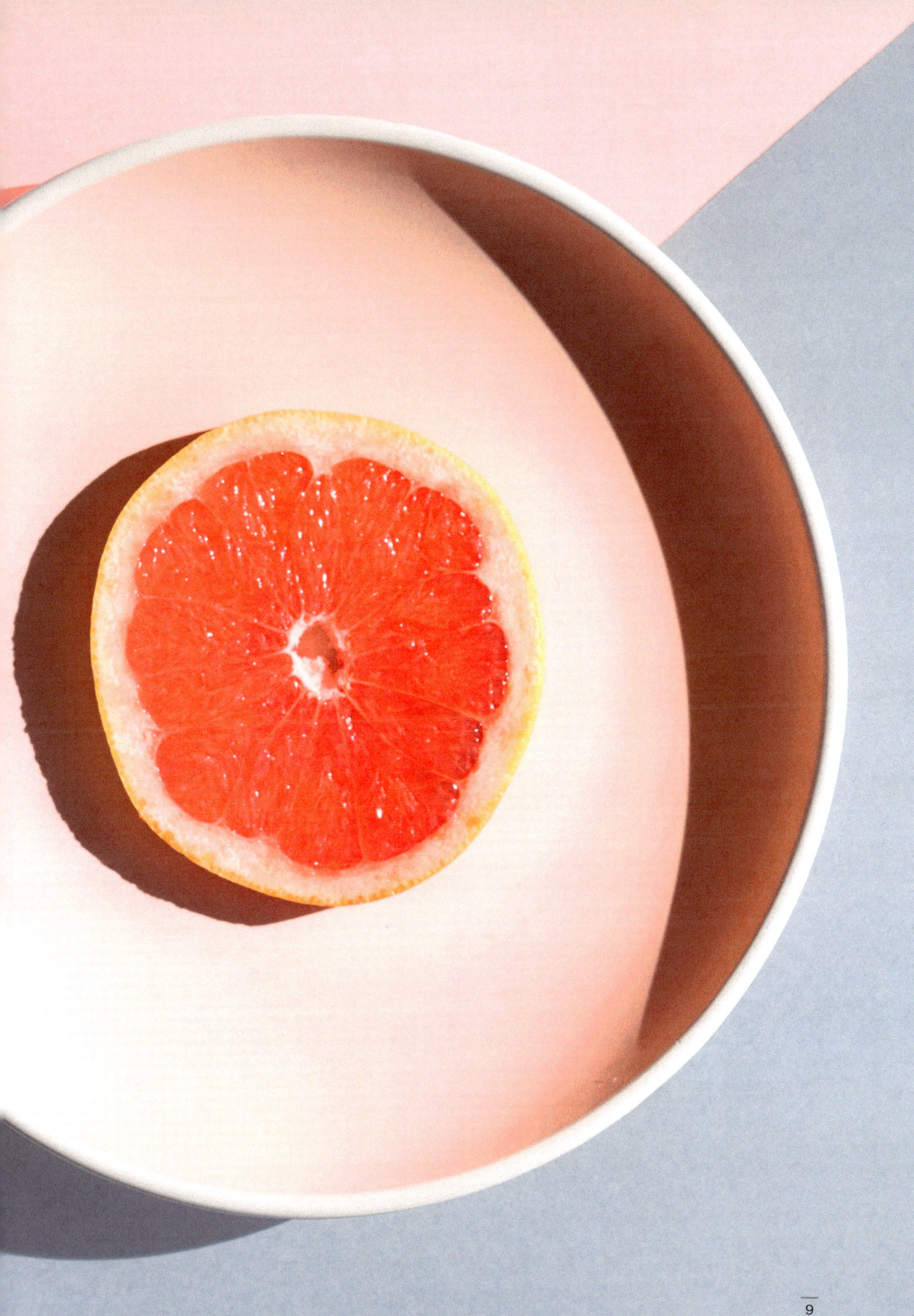

one hand, it tracked with widespread beliefs about weight loss: the workouts were punishing and the diets restrictive, so it stood to reason that the men and women on the show would slim down. Still, 20 pounds in a week was a lot. To understand how they were doing it, he decided to study 14 of the contestants for a scientific paper.

Hall quickly learned that in reality-TV land, a week doesn't always translate into a precise seven days, but no matter: the weight being lost was real, speedy and huge. Over the course of the season, the contestants lost an average of 127 pounds each and about 64% of their body fat. If his study could uncover what was happening in their bodies on a physiological level, he thought, maybe he'd be able to help the staggering 71% of American adults who are overweight.

What he didn't expect to learn was that even when the conditions for weight loss are TV-perfect—with a tough but motivating trainer, strict meal plans and killer workouts—the body will, in the long run, fight like hell to get that fat back. Over time, 13 of the 14 contestants Hall studied gained, on average, 66% of the weight they'd lost on the show, and four became heavier than they were before the competition.

That may be depressing enough to make even the most motivated dieter give up. "There's this notion of 'Why bother trying?' " says Hall. But finding answers to the weight-loss puzzle has never been more critical. The vast majority of American adults are overweight; nearly 40% are clinically obese. And doctors now know that excess body fat dramatically increases the risk of serious health problems, including Type 2 diabetes, heart disease, depression, respiratory problems, major cancers and even fertility problems. A 2017 study found that obesity now drives more early preventable deaths in the U.S. than smoking. This has fueled a weight-loss industry worth $72 billion, selling everything from diet pills to meal plans to fancy gym memberships.

It's also fueled a rise in research. In fiscal 2019 the NIH will spend an estimated $995 million in funding for obesity research, including Hall's, and that research is giving scientists a new understanding of why dieting is so hard, why keeping the weight off over time is even harder and why the prevailing wisdom about weight loss seems to work only sometimes—and for only some people.

What scientists are uncovering should bring fresh hope to the 155 million Americans who are overweight, according to the U.S. Centers for Disease Control and Prevention. Leading researchers finally agree, for instance, that exercise, while critical to good health, on its own is not an especially reliable way to lose weight. And the overly simplistic arithmetic of calories in vs. calories out has given way to the more nuanced understanding that it's the composition of a person's diet—rather than how much of it they can burn off working out—that sustains weight loss.

The researchers also know that the best diet for you is very likely not the best diet for your next-door neighbor. Individual responses to different diets—from low-fat and vegan to low-carb and Paleo—vary enormously. "Some people on a diet program lose 60 pounds and keep it off for two years, and other people follow the same program religiously and they gain five pounds," says Frank Sacks, a weight-loss researcher and professor of cardiovascular disease prevention at the Harvard T.H. Chan School of Public Health. "If we can figure out why, the potential to help people will be huge."

Hall, Sacks and other scientists are showing that the key to weight loss appears to be highly personalized rather than the adoption of trendy diets. And although weight loss will never be easy for anyone, the evidence is mounting that it's possible for anyone to reach a healthy weight—people just need to find their best way there.

Dieting has been an American preoccupation since long before the obesity epidemic took off in the 1980s. In the 1830s, Presbyterian minister Sylvester Graham touted a vegetarian diet that excluded spices, condiments and alcohol. At the turn of the 20th century, it was fashionable to chew food until it was liquefied, sometimes up to 722 times before

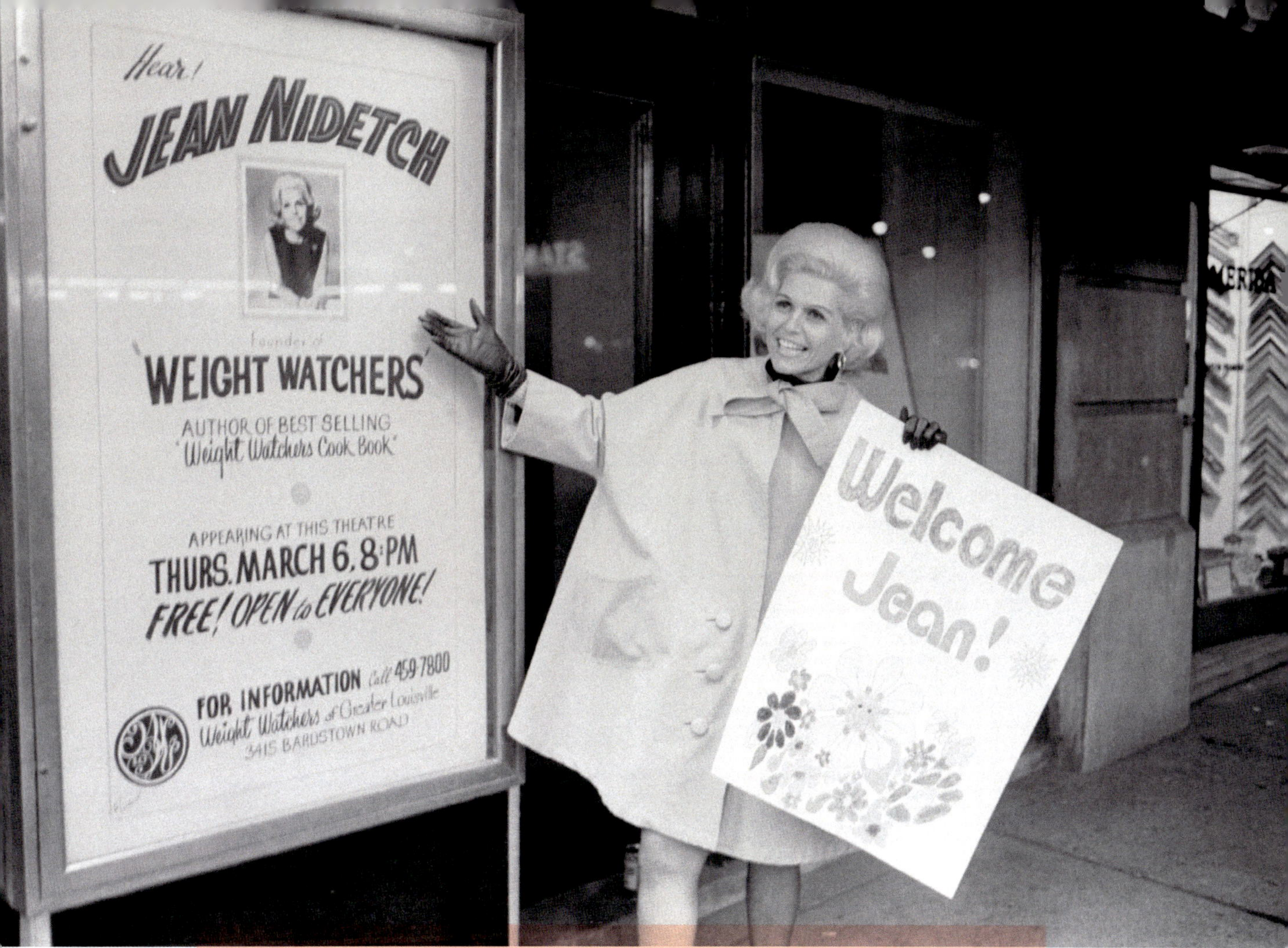

Jean Nidetch—who co-founded Weight Watchers after succeeding at losing a lot of weight with support from friends—before giving a speech in Louisville, Ky., in 1969

swallowing, based on the advice of a popular nutrition expert named Horace Fletcher. Lore has it that at about the same time, President William Howard Taft adopted a fairly contemporary plan—low-fat, low-calorie, with a daily food log—after he got stuck in a White House bathtub.

The concept of the calorie as a unit of energy had been studied and shared in scientific circles throughout Europe for some time, but it wasn't until World War I that calorie counting became de rigueur in the U.S. Amid global food shortages, the American government needed a way to encourage people to cut back on their food intake, so it issued its first-ever "scientific diet" for Americans, which had calorie counting at its core.

In the following decades, when being rail-thin became ever more desirable, nearly all dieting advice stressed meals that were low in calories. There was the grapefruit diet of the 1930s (in which people ate half a grapefruit with every meal out of a belief that the fruit contained fat-burning enzymes) and the cabbage-soup diet of the 1950s (a flatulence-inducing plan in which people ate cabbage soup every day for a week alongside low-calorie meals).

Birth of a diet boom

The 1960s saw the beginning of the massive commercialization of dieting in the U.S. That's when a New York housewife named Jean Nidetch began hosting friends at her home to talk about their issues with weight and dieting. Nidetch was a self-proclaimed cookie lover who had struggled for years to slim down. Her weekly meetings helped her so much—she lost 72 pounds in about a year—that she ultimately turned those living-room gatherings into a company called Weight Watchers. When it went public in 1968, she and her co-founders became

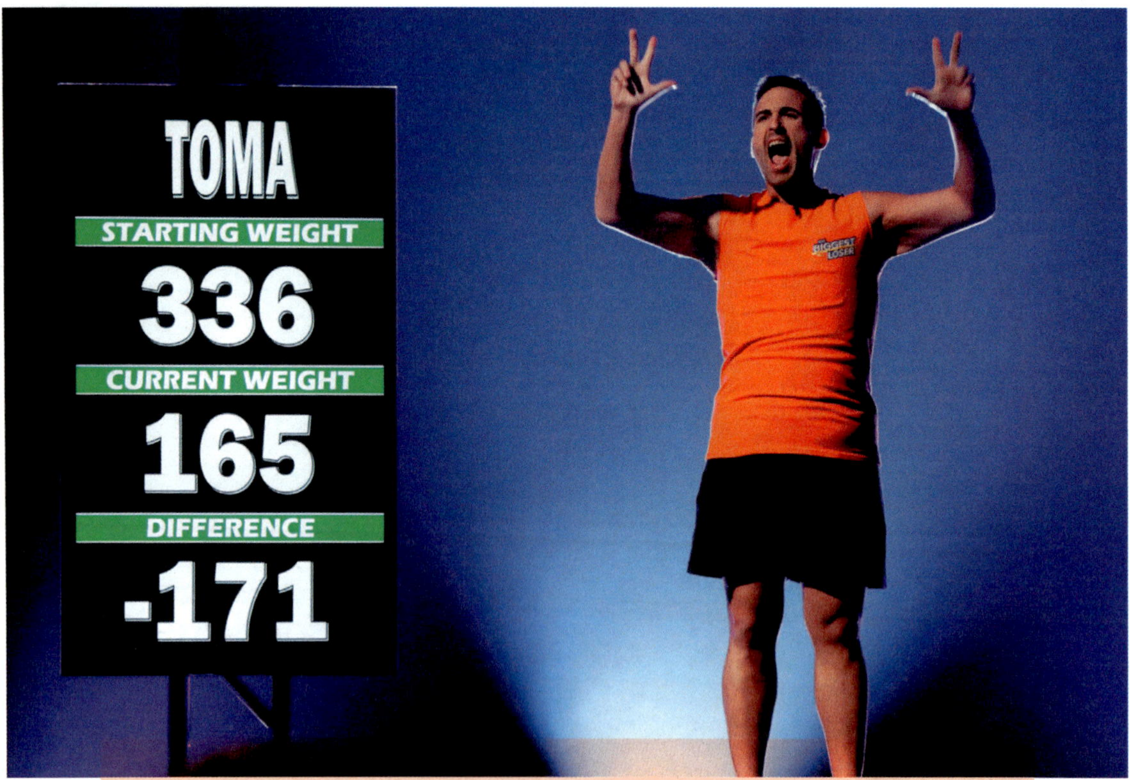

The 2016 live finale of The Biggest Loser. *The series fueled Americans' interest in wellness—and helped scientists better understand why it's hard to keep weight off.*

millionaires overnight. Nearly half a century later, Weight Watchers, which in 2018 was rebranded WW (with the slogan "Wellness That Works"), remains one of the most commercially successful diet companies in the world, with 3.9 million active users and $1.5 billion in revenue in 2018.

What most of these diets had in common was an idea that is still popular today: eat less fattening food and you will lose weight. Even the low-fat craze that kicked off in the late 1970s—which was based on the intuitively appealing but incorrect notion that eating fat will make you fat—depended on the calorie-counting model of weight loss.

That's not what happened when people went low-fat, though. The diet trend coincided with weight *gain*. In 1990, adults with obesity made up less than 15% of the U.S. population. By 2010, most states were reporting obesity in 25% or more of their populations. Today that has swelled to 40% of the adult population. For kids and teens, it's 18.5%.

Research like Hall's is beginning to explain why. As demoralizing as his initial findings were, they weren't altogether surprising: more than 80% of people with obesity who lose weight gain it back. That's because when you lose weight, your resting metabolism (how much energy your body uses when at rest) slows down—possibly an evolutionary holdover from the days when food scarcity was common.

What Hall discovered, however—and what frankly startled him—was that even when the *Biggest Loser* contestants gained back some of their weight, their resting metabolism didn't speed up along with it. Instead, in a cruel twist, it remained low, burning about 700 fewer calories per day than it did before they started losing weight in the first place. "When people see the slowing metabolism numbers," says Hall, "their eyes bulge like, 'How is that even possible?' "

The contestants lose a massive amount of weight in a relatively short period of time—not how most doctors recommend you lose weight—but research shows that the same slowing metabolism Hall observed tends to happen to regular Joes too. Most people who lose weight gain back the pounds they lost at a rate of two to four pounds per year.

For the 2.2 billion people around the world who are overweight, Hall's findings can seem like a formula for failure—and, at the same time, vindication. They show that it's indeed biology, not a lack of willpower, that makes it so hard to lose weight. The findings also make it seem as if the body itself will sabotage any effort to keep weight off in the long term.

But a slower metabolism is not the full story. There are many people who succeed in losing weight and keeping it off. Hall has seen it happen more times than he can count. The catch is that some people appear to succeed with almost every diet approach—it just varies from person to person.

"You take a bunch of people and randomly assign them to follow a low-carb diet or a low-fat diet," Hall says. "You follow them for a couple of years, and what you tend to see is that average weight loss is almost no different between the two groups as a whole. But within each group, there are people who are very successful, people who don't lose any weight and people who gain weight."

Understanding what it is about a given diet that works for a given person remains the holy grail of weight-loss science. But experts are getting closer.

For the past 25 years, Rena Wing, a professor of psychiatry and human behavior at Brown University, has run the National Weight Control Registry (NWCR) as a way to track people who successfully lose weight and keep it off. "When we started it, the perspective was that almost no one succeeded at losing weight and keeping it off," says James O. Hill, Wing's collaborator and an obesity researcher at the University of Colorado. "We didn't believe that was the case, but we didn't know for sure because we didn't have the data."

To qualify for initial inclusion in the registry, a person must have lost at least 30 pounds and maintained that weight loss for a year or longer. Today the registry includes more than 10,000 people from across the 50 states with an average weight loss of 66 pounds per person. On average, people on the current list have kept their weight off for more than five years.

When you lose weight, your resting metabolism—the amount of energy your body uses when at rest—slows down.

The most revealing detail about the registry: everyone on the list has lost significant amounts of weight—but in different ways. About 45% of them say they lost weight following various diets on their own, for instance, and 55% say they used a structured weight-loss program. And most of them had to try more than one diet before the weight loss stuck.

What keeps weight off

The researchers have identified some similarities among them: 98% of the people in the study say they modified their diet in some way, with most cutting back on how much they ate in a given day. Another through line: 94% increased their physical activity, and the most popular form of exercise was walking.

"There's nothing magical about what they do," says Wing. "Some people emphasize exercise more than others, some follow low-carb diets and some follow low-fat diets. The one commonality is that they had to make changes in their everyday behaviors."

When asked how they've kept the weight off, the vast majority of people in the study say they eat breakfast every day, weigh themselves at least once a week, watch less than 10 hours of television per week and exercise about an hour a day, on average.

The researchers have also looked at their attitudes and behavior. They found that most of them do not consider themselves type A, dispelling the idea that only obsessive superplanners can stick to a diet. They learned that many successful dieters are self-described morning people. (Other research supports the anecdotal: for some reason, night owls tend to weigh more than larks.) The researchers also noticed that people with long-term weight loss tended to be motivated by something other than a slimmer waist—like a health scare or the desire to live a longer life, to be able to spend more time with loved ones.

Finding your fit

The researchers at the NWCR say it's unlikely that the people they study are somehow genetically endowed or blessed with a personality that makes weight loss easy for them. After all, most people in the study say they had failed several times before when they had tried to lose weight. Instead they were highly motivated, and they kept trying different things until they found something that worked for them.

"Losing weight and keeping it off is hard, and if anyone tells you it's easy, run the other way," says Hill. "But it is absolutely possible, and when people do it, their lives are changed for the better." (Hill came under fire in 2015 for his role as president of an obesity think tank funded by Coca-Cola and stepped down. During his tenure, the NWCR published one paper with partial funding from Coca-Cola; the researchers say their study wasn't influenced by that financial support.)

Hill, Wing and their colleagues agree that perhaps the most encouraging lesson to be gleaned from their registry is the simplest: in a group of 10,000 real-life biggest losers, no two people lost the weight in quite the same way.

"Losing weight and keeping it off is hard. But it is absolutely possible, and when people do it, their lives are changed for the better."

The Bariatric Medical Institute in Ottawa is founded on that thinking. When people enroll in its weight-loss program, they all start on the same six-month diet and exercise plan—but they are encouraged to diverge from the program, with the help of a physician, whenever they want, in order to figure out what works best for them. The program takes a whole-person approach to weight loss, which means that behavior, psychology and budget—not just biology—inform each person's plan.

"We have a plan that involves getting enough calories and protein and so forth, but we are not married to it," says Yoni Freedhoff, an obesity expert and the medical director of the clinic. "We try to understand where people are struggling, and then we adjust. Everyone here is doing things slightly differently."

In most cases, people try a few different plans before they get it right. Jody Jeans, an IT project manager in Ottawa, had been overweight since she was a child. When she came to the clinic in 2007, she was 5 feet 4 inches tall and weighed 240 pounds. Though she had lost weight in her 20s doing Weight Watchers, she gained it back after she lost a job and the stress led her to overeat. Jeans would wake up on a Monday and decide she was starting a diet, or never eating dessert again, only to scrap the plan a couple of days, if not hours, later. "Unless you've had a lot of weight to lose, you don't understand what it's like," she says. "It's overwhelming, and people look at you like it's your fault."

A March 2017 study found that people who internalize weight stigma have a harder time maintaining weight loss. That's why most experts argue that pushing people toward health goals rather than a number on the scale can yield better results. "When you solely focus on weight, you may give up on changes in your life that would have positive benefits," says the NIH's Hall.

It took Jeans five years to lose 75 pounds while on a program at Freedhoff's institute, but by paying attention to portion sizes, writing down all her meals and eating more frequent, smaller meals throughout the day, she's kept the weight off for an additional seven years. She credits the slow, steady pace for her success. Though she's never been especially motivated to exercise, she found it helpful to track her food each day as well as make sure she ate enough filling protein and fiber—without having to rely on bland diet staples like grilled chicken over greens (hold the dressing). "I'm a foodie," Jeans says. "If you told me I had to eat the same things every day, it would be torture."

Natalie Casagrande was on the same program that Jeans was on, but Freedhoff and his colleagues used a different approach with her. Casagrande's weight had fluctuated throughout her life, and she had attempted dangerous diets like starving herself. One time, she even dropped from a size 14 to a size 0 in just a few months. When she signed up for the program, Casagrande weighed 173 pounds. At 4 feet

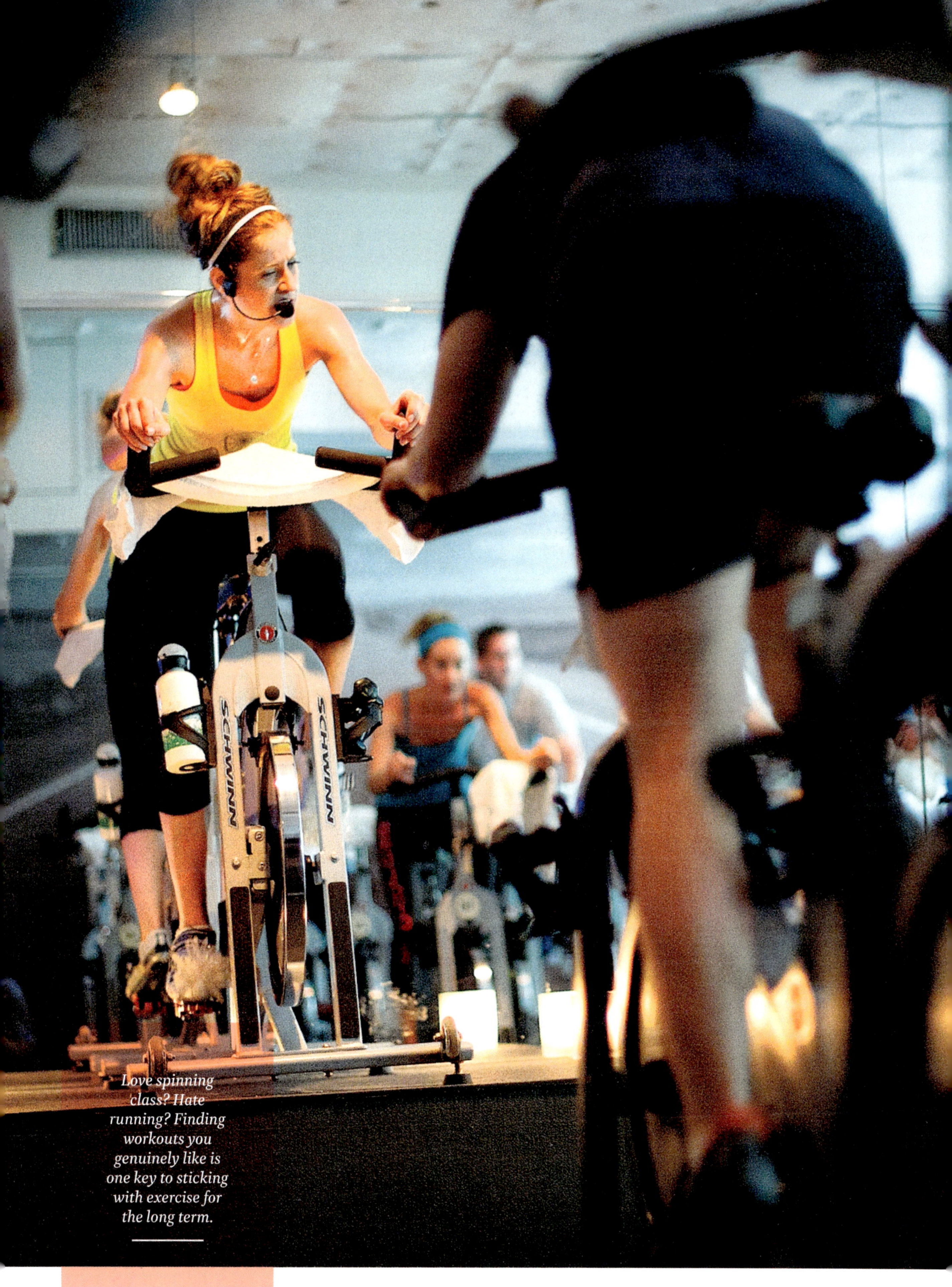

Love spinning class? Hate running? Finding workouts you genuinely like is one key to sticking with exercise for the long term.

11 inches, that meant she was clinically obese, which means having a body mass index of 30 or more.

Once she started working with the team at the Bariatric Medical Institute, Casagrande also tracked her food, but unlike Jeans, she never enjoyed the process. What she did love was exercise. She found her workouts motivating. By meeting with the clinic's psychologist, she also learned that she had generalized anxiety, which helped explain her bouts of emotional eating.

It took Casagrande three tries over three years before she finally lost substantial weight. During one relapse period, she gained 10 pounds. She tweaked her plan to focus more on cooking and managing her mental health and tried again. She reached 116 pounds and has maintained that weight ever since. "It takes a lot of trial and error to figure out what works," she says. "Not every day is going to be perfect, but I'm here because I pushed through the bad days."

Genes and gut bacteria

Freedhoff says that learning which variables are most important for each person—be they psychological or food-based—matters more to him than identifying one diet that works for everyone. "So long as we continue to pigeonhole people into certain diets without considering the individuals, the more likely we are to run into problems," he says. That's why a significant portion of his meetings with patients is spent talking about the person's daily duties, their socioeconomic status, their mental health, their comfort in the kitchen. "Unfortunately," he says, "that's not the norm. The amount of effort needed to understand your patients is more than many doctors put in."

Exactly why weight loss can vary so much for people on the same diet plan still eludes scientists. "It's the biggest open question in the field," says the NIH's Hall. "I wish I knew the answer."

Some speculate it's people's genetics. Over the past several years, researchers have identified nearly 100 genetic markers that appear to be linked to being obese or being overweight, and there's no doubt genes play an important role in how some people break down calories and store fat. But experts estimate that obesity-related genes account for just 3% of the differences between people's sizes—and those same genes that predispose people to weight gain existed 30 years ago, and 100 years ago, suggesting that genes alone cannot explain the rapid rise in obesity.

What's more, a recent study of 9,000 people found that whether a person carried a gene variation associated with weight gain had no influence on that person's ability to lose weight. "We think this is good news," says study author John Mathers, a professor of human nutrition at Newcastle University. "Carrying the high-risk form of the gene makes you more likely to be a bit heavier, but it shouldn't prevent you from losing weight."

Another hot area of research is the link between weight gain and chemicals we are exposed to every day—substances like the bisphenol A (BPA) found in linings of canned goods and cash-register receipts, the flame retardants in sofas and mattresses, the pesticide residues on our food and the phthalates found in plastics and cosmetics. What these chemicals have in common is their ability to mimic human hormones, and some scientists worry that they may be wreaking havoc on the delicate endocrine system, driving fat storage.

Experts estimate that obesity-related genes account for just 3% of the differences between people's sizes.

"The old paradigm was that poor diet and lack of exercise are underpinning obesity, but now we understand that chemical exposures are an important third factor in the origin of the obesity epidemic," says Leonardo Trasande, an associate professor of pediatrics, environmental medicine and population health at New York University's School of Medicine. "Chemicals can disrupt hormones and metabolism, which can contribute to disease and disability."

Scientists are also exploring how the microbiome—the trillions of bacteria that live inside and on the surface of the human body—may be influencing how the body metabolizes what we eat. Eran Elinav and Eran Segal, researchers for the Personalized Nutrition Project at the Weizmann Institute of Science in Israel, believe the variation in diet success may lie in the way our microbiomes react to foods.

In a 2015 study, Elinav and Segal gave 800 men and

women devices that measured their blood-sugar levels every five minutes for a one-week period. The participants filled out questionnaires about their health, provided blood and stool samples and had their microbiomes sequenced. They also used a mobile app to keep track of their food intake, sleep and exercise.

The researchers found that blood-sugar levels varied widely among people after they ate, even when they ate the exact same meal. This suggests that umbrella recommendations for how to eat could be meaningless. "It was a major surprise to us," says Segal.

The researchers developed an algorithm for each person in the trial using the data they had gathered and found that they could accurately predict a person's blood-sugar response to a given food on the basis of their microbiome. That's why Elinav and Segal believe the next frontier in weight-loss science lies in the gut; they believe their algorithm could ultimately help doctors prescribe highly specific diets for people according to how they respond to foods.

Unsurprisingly, there are businesses trying to cash in on this idea. Online supplement companies already hawk personalized probiotic pills, with testimonials from customers claiming they lost weight taking them. So far, research to support the probiotic-pill approach to weight loss is scant. Ditto the genetic tests that claim to be able to tell you whether you're better off on a low-carb diet or a vegan one.

When people are asked to envision their perfect size, many cite a dream weight loss up to three times as great as what a doctor might recommend. Given how difficult that can be to pull off, it's no surprise so many people give up trying to lose weight altogether.

But most of us do not need to lose quite so much weight to improve our health. With just a 5% to 10% loss of weight, people will experience changes in blood pressure and blood-sugar control, lowering their risk for heart disease and Type 2 diabetes.

For Ottawa's Jeans, recalibrating her expectations is what helped her finally lose weight in a healthy—and sustainable—way. People may look at her and see someone who could still afford to lose a few pounds, she says, but she's proud of her weight, and she is well within the range of what a good doctor would call healthy. "You have to accept that you're never going to be a willowy model," she says. "But I am at a very good weight that I can manage." ☐

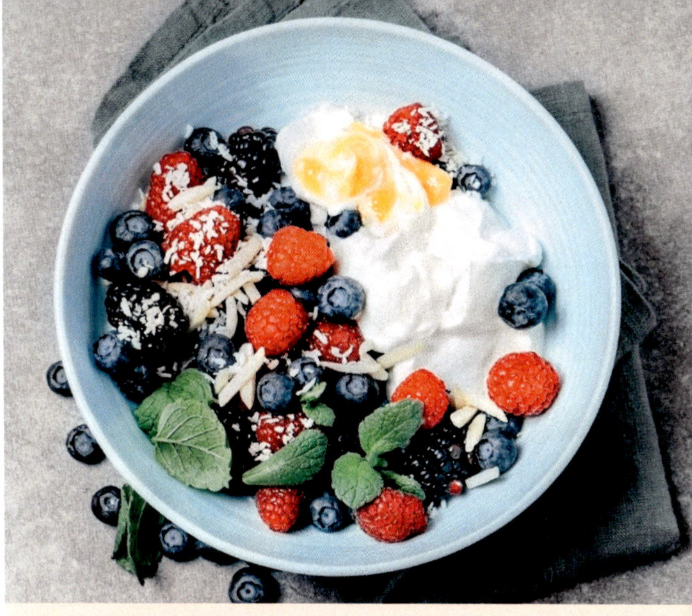

5 SECRETS TO LASTING LOSS

This is what we know about successful dieters from the National Weight Control Registry

They eat breakfast. » People in the NWCR have lost at least 30 pounds and kept it off for at least a year. One habit they share: they have a morning meal every day. Research suggests this is a healthy strategy for controlling insulin and jump-starting your metabolism.

They exercise every day. » What else do we know about the successful losers in the NWCR, many of whom have kept the pounds away for five years or longer? They move a lot after losing weight, exercising for about an hour a day on average. A common exercise is walking. When it comes to walking or running, you get a benefit whether you do 60 minutes at once or break it into 15- or 20-minute chunks.

They trim TV time. » The long-term losers in the NWCR watch less than 10 hours of television a week. That's more time for walking.

They do scales. » By weighing themselves about once a week, they give themselves the chance to make tweaks to their eating and exercise if their weight starts to creep up.

They have a deeper goal. » Identifying an intrinsic goal helps dieters succeed long-term. People who have achieved lasting weight loss often have a hope beyond looking slim—whether it's to live longer, to avoid chronic health problems or to have energy to keep up with children or grandchildren.

What Is Intermittent Fasting and Is It Actually Good for You?

Researchers are learning that eating very little food two days a week leads to lasting weight loss, reduced risk of diabetes and other health benefits

› **By Markham Heid**

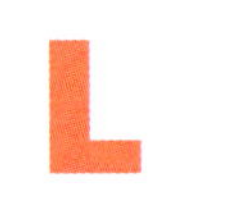

ASTING WEIGHT LOSS. PROTECTION FROM DIABETES, heart disease and cancer. Improved brain health. Enhanced physical fitness. It seems as if every week, researchers turn up a new benefit associated with intermittent fasting: eating schedules that incorporate regular periods of low or no food consumption.

By eating normally several days a week and eating much less on the others, a person may be able to shift his or her body's cellular and metabolic processes in ways that promote optimal health. And experts say that while many blanks still need to be filled in, some of the positive health effects of intermittent fasting are no longer in doubt.

"There continues to be good evidence that intermittent fasting is producing weight-loss benefits, and we also have some evidence that these diets can reduce inflammation, they can reduce blood pressure and resting heart rate, and they seem to have

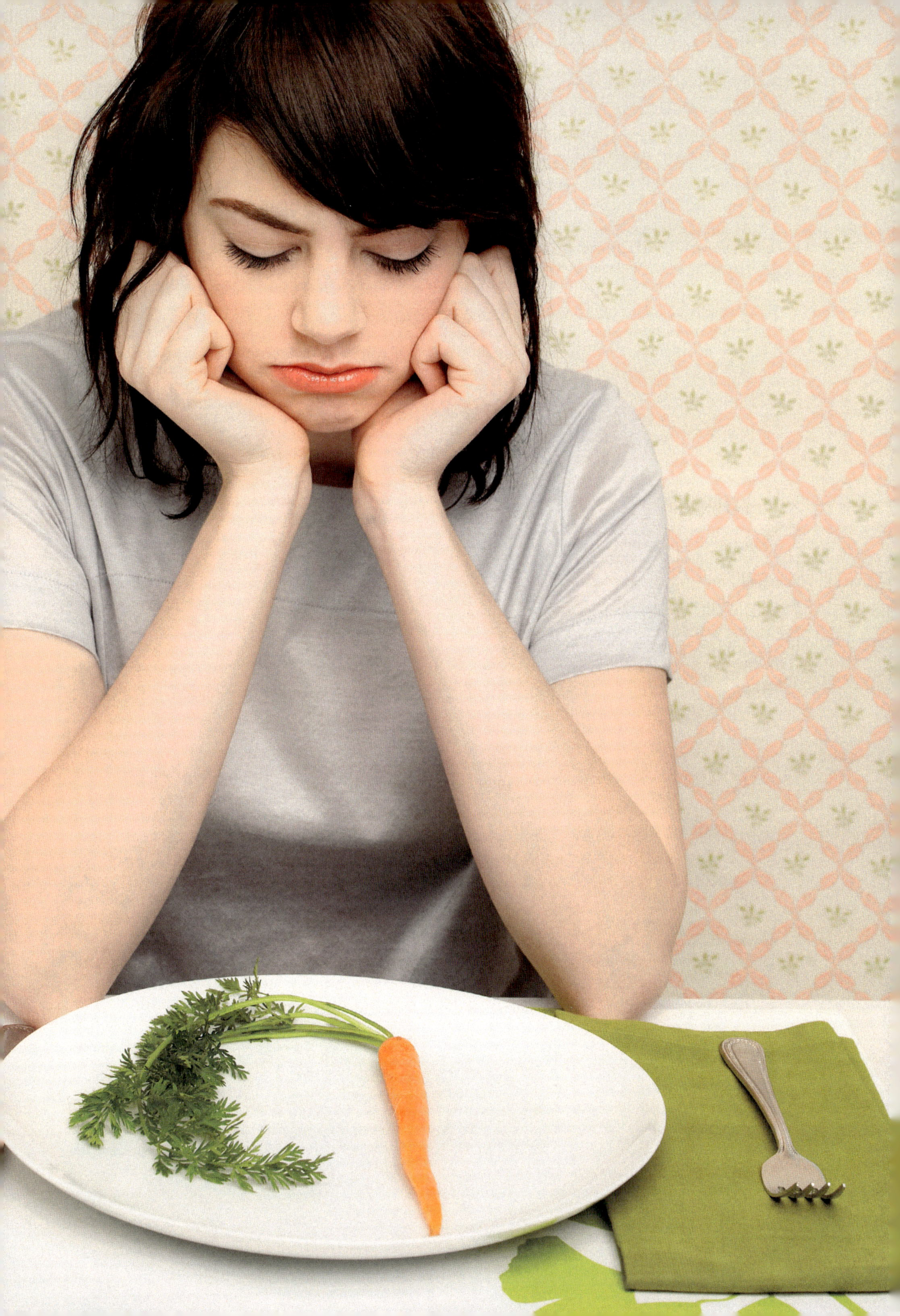

beneficial effects on the cardiovascular system," says Benjamin Horne, director of cardiovascular and genetic epidemiology at Utah's nonprofit Intermountain Healthcare system, who has published research on the subject. "[Intermittent fasting] is something that is moving into practice in the medical field, and it's a reasonable approach for people who don't like daily restriction of their calories."

The bulk of the early research on fasting focused on weight loss. Studies comparing intermittent fasting (also known as intermittent energy restriction) with calorie-cutting diets have found that people lose more weight on fasting plans. They also seem to like the diet better; intermittent fasters tend to drop out of dietary studies at lower rates than calorie cutters.

"Intermittent fasting is a good option for weight loss for overweight and obese people," says Michelle Harvie, a research dietitian with the Prevent Breast Cancer unit at the Manchester Breast Centre in the U.K. Harvie has co-authored studies on intermittent fasting, and her research has repeatedly shown that it outperforms traditional diets in weight loss, reduction of body fat and improvement in insulin resistance. She's also found some evidence that intermittent fasting may beat traditional weight-loss plans in lowering women's risk for breast cancer.

Intermittent fasters seem to like the diet; they drop out of dietary studies at lower rates than calorie cutters.

Most of Harvie's research has examined 5:2 fasting plans—restricting calorie intake two days a week while allowing normal eating the other five. But she says there's also promising research on diets that impose fasting every other day (usually referred to as alternate-day fasting plans) and on time-restricted fasting, in which daily food consumption is restricted to a six- or eight-hour window.

"None of these have been studied head-to-head, but they all improve health," says Mark Mattson, chief of the Laboratory of Neurosciences at the National Institute on Aging and a professor of neuroscience at the Johns Hopkins School of Medicine. Mattson has published multiple studies on intermittent fasting. There's evidence these diets bolster stress resistance and combat inflammation at a cellular level, he says. "People undergo a metabolic switch in which the liver's energy stores are depleted, and so the body's cells start using fat and ketones for energy," he explains. This switch is a form of mild challenge to the human body that he compares to exercise; just as running or lifting weights stresses the body in beneficial ways, the stress imposed by fasting appears to induce some similarly beneficial adaptations. Whether you're talking about physical activity or fasting, "these cycles of challenge, recovery, challenge, recovery seem to optimize both function and durability of most cell sites," he says.

Fasting also makes sense evolutionarily. All-the-time access to food is a relatively new phenomenon in human history. Back when sustenance was harder to come by, "natural selection would have favored individuals whose brains and bodies functioned well in a food-deprived state," Mattson says.

But experts acknowledge there are still unknowns. Almost all the human research to date has been in overweight or obese adults. "We don't know of its benefits in normal-weight people, as it has not been studied," Harvie says. It's also not yet clear if there are any long-term risks.

How should you try it? Mattson says the 5:2 plan has the most data backing it up. For two days a week (either consecutive or broken up), consume just 500 daily calories of fat or protein—foods like eggs, fish and nuts. One day's meal plan could be two scrambled eggs for breakfast (180 calories), a quarter cup of almonds for a snack (200 calories) and a four-ounce cod fillet for dinner (100 calories). You can divvy up calories however you like. "But better to have no or very little carbohydrates," he says. While you'll want to eat healthy foods the rest of the week, you won't have to count calories or avoid carbs.

He says you can expect to feel hungry for the first few weeks. "But by the end of the first month, we've found, almost everyone has adapted and there are no symptoms," he says. It may eventually turn out that longer periods of fasting—say, going 24 hours without any food at all—could be even more beneficial. But more human data is needed.

"I suggest people talk to their physician first," Horne stresses, adding that intermittent fasting is not a silver bullet: "There's no amount of exercise or fasting that can overcome a bad diet or an unhealthy lifestyle." □

FADS: THE GOOD, THE BAD, THE RIDICULOUS

A brief history of weight loss and body positivity **BY EMILY JOSHU**

1810–1820s: Vinegar and Water Diet » Romantic-era poet Lord Byron believed that obesity causes lethargy and stupidity, so he hopped onto the Vinegar and Water Diet, according to the book *Calories and Corsets*. It's as appetizing as it sounds: water mixed with apple-cider vinegar. And to the present day, some people claim this method burns fat.

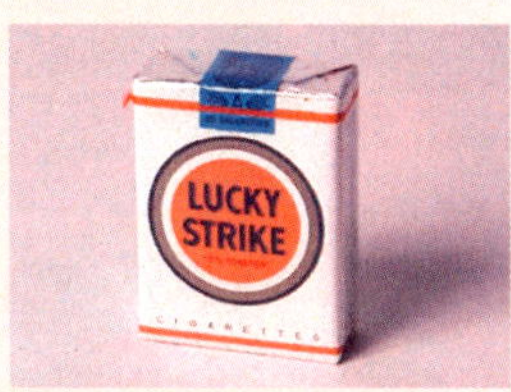

1925: Cigarette Diet » The roaring '20s introduced its own dubious diet plan: smoke your way slim. A Lucky Strike cigarette ad campaign advised to "reach for a Lucky instead of a sweet" and "to keep a slender figure . . . reach for a Lucky." It's hard to imagine any advice worse than that.

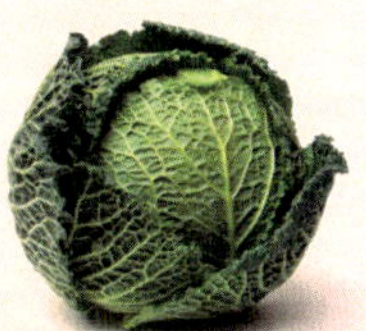

1950s: Cabbage-Soup Diet » This plan promised you could lose 10 pounds in seven days by living largely on—you guessed it—cabbage soup. (On certain days you could eat things like apples and beef.) Reality check: any more than one or two pounds of lost weight per week is water weight, not fat.

1963: TaB debuts » It wasn't the first diet soda (Dr Pepper had one a year earlier), but Coca-Cola's TaB was the first diet drink to hit big. Although TaB is still on the market today, diet-soda sales in general have fizzled, as science has shown diet soda can actually trick your body into craving sugar.

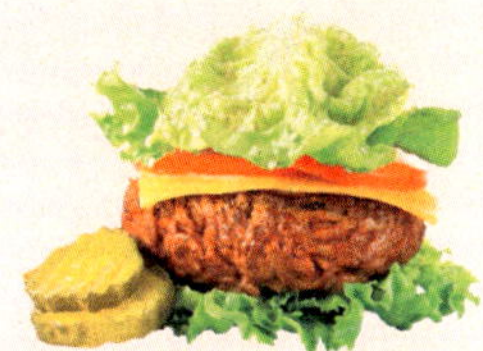

1972: The Atkins Diet catches on » The high-protein-diet craze began with the publication of a book called *Dr. Atkins' Diet Revolution*. Atkins—a cardiologist—preached that severely limiting carbs causes the body to burn fat. While his diet is still popular, most experts recommend a more moderate approach to limiting simple carbs.

2004: *The Biggest Loser* makes weight loss must-see TV » As America became more health conscious, *The Biggest Loser* made riveting TV out of facing off to get fit. The show—criticized for encouraging contestants to lose weight too fast—lasted 17 seasons and made household names out of Jillian Michaels and Bob Harper.

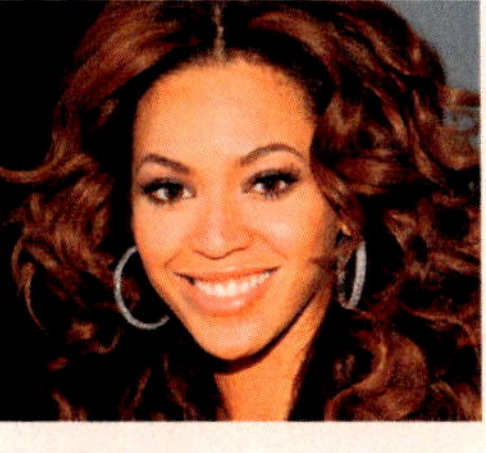

2006: Beyoncé and the Master Cleanse » To lose 20 pounds fast for the movie *Dreamgirls*, Beyoncé reportedly went on the Lemonade Diet (foreshadowing, perhaps?). Also known as the Master Cleanse, it involves downing a concoction of hot water, lemon juice, maple syrup and cayenne pepper several times a day, plus a laxative tea at night. Not a recipe for healthy, lasting weight loss.

2010s: Paleo Diet » In his book *The Paleo Diet*, Dr. Loren Cordain urged people to stick with Paleolithic-era food groups—meat, seafood, fruits and vegetables—and skip foods created through modern farming practices, like grains and dairy products. This diet has been criticized for eliminating grains, which are high-fiber and linked to weight loss.

2009: The dad bod » Describing a man in married-life mode and "softly round," the term "dad bod" made it into the Urban Dictionary in 2009. The sobriquet's popularity suggests that men get judged for their bodies too—and that there is something appealing about a more realistic, attainable physique.

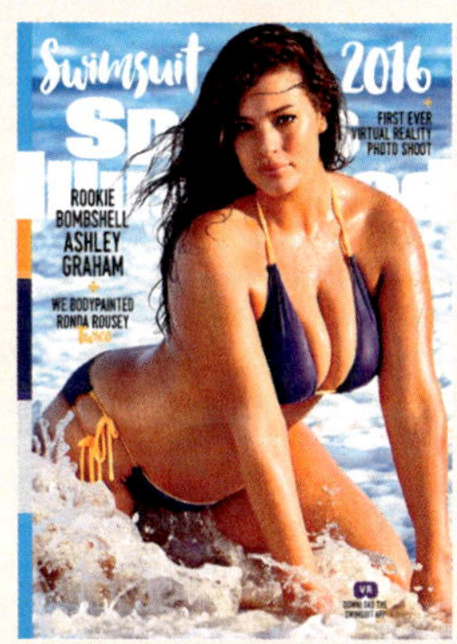

2016: Ashley Graham graces the *Sports Illustrated* cover » People of all sizes cheered when Ashley Graham—a stunning, fit size-16 model—appeared on the cover of *Sports Illustrated*'s swimsuit issue. She also landed fashion-magazine covers, reminding the world that beauty is not one-size-fits-all.

2018: Weight Watchers becomes WW » As fewer Americans go on diets, Weight Watchers rebranded itself as WW with the slogan "Wellness That Works."

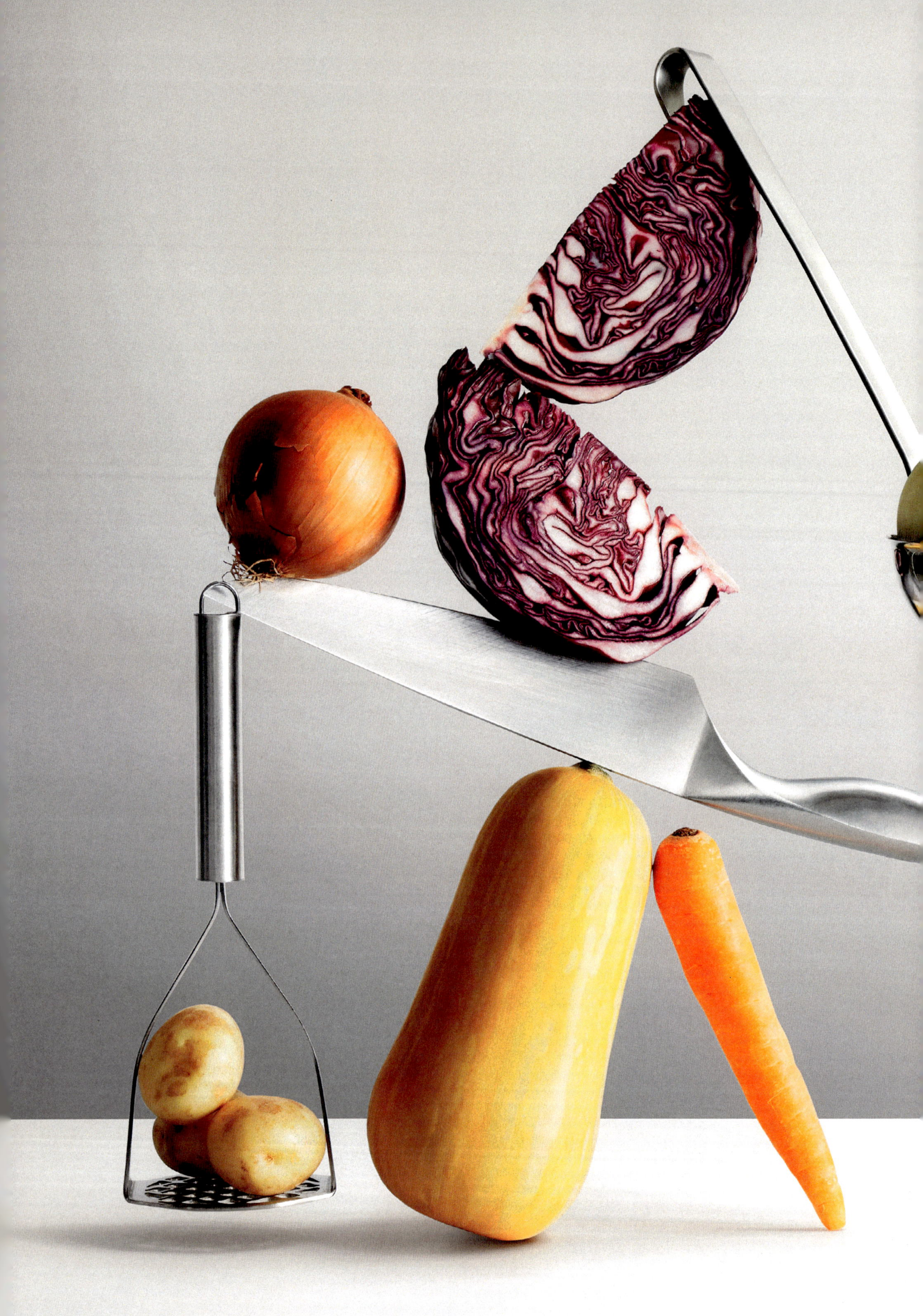

Why You Should Stop Counting Calories

Eating more of the right foods and cutting back on added sugar help the body naturally regulate weight, according to the latest thinking

› ***By Mandy Oaklander***

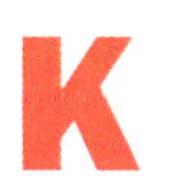

KERI RABE, AN ELEMENTARY-SCHOOL LIBRARIAN IN Austin, Texas, used to be a hard-core calorie counter. Each day for a year, she logged everything she ate. She would only eat favorites like twice-baked potatoes and tater-tot casseroles if she made them with low-fat dairy, believing dietary fat would make her fat. She calculated every last calorie. "I thought for sure that was the only way to consistently lose weight," she says. "I thought I'd have to do it for the rest of my life."

By one measure, it worked; Rabe lost 10 pounds that year. But even though she met her goal, she was frustrated. She hated doing math before and after every meal, and even though she got away with eating low-quality food while losing weight, she still didn't feel good—and she wasn't satisfied.

So one day, Rabe stopped logging and went searching for a better path, not just to lose weight but to keep it off. "I was looking for a way I could eat for the rest of my life," she says.

Rabe was about to learn what many experts are discovering: that the quality of calories rather than the quantity is what matters most for staying healthy, losing weight and maintaining those results.

"When you eat the right quality and balance of foods, your body can do the rest on its own," says David Ludwig, an endocrinologist, researcher and professor at Harvard Medical School, who wrote the 2016 weight-loss book *Always Hungry?* "You don't have to count calories or go by the numbers."

The problem with foods that make people fat isn't that they have too many calories, says Ludwig. It's that they cause a cascade of reactions in the body that promote fat storage and make us overeat. Processed carbohydrates—foods like chips, cookies, soda, crackers and even white rice—digest quickly into sugar and increase levels of the hormone insulin.

"Insulin is like Miracle-Gro for your fat cells," explains Ludwig. It directs cells to snap up calories in the blood and store them as fat, leaving the body feeling hungry in a hurry. This is why it's so easy to devour a big bag of chips or a blueberry muffin and still feel famished.

Repeat this cycle too many times and your metabolism will start working against you. What's more, "when humans try to reduce their calorie balance, the body fights back," says Ludwig. This happens in two ways: the body's metabolism slows in order to keep calories around longer, and you begin to feel hungrier. "This combination of rising hunger and slowing metabolism is a battle that we're destined to lose over the long term," he adds.

Replace processed carbs with healthy fats. Fats don't raise insulin, so they can be a key ally for weight loss, says David Ludwig.

Put fat back on the plate

The best way to break this fattening cycle is to replace processed carbs with healthy fats, Ludwig points out: "Fats don't raise insulin at all, so they can be a key ally for weight loss."

That idea, of course, contradicts decades of dietary advice. Americans have long been warned about the dangers of fat, since the nutrient contains more than twice as many calories as carbohydrates and proteins. By the math alone, replacing fat with carbs seems like a good idea—but it's not. Studies have shown that people on a low-fat diet tend to lose less weight than people on a low-carbohydrate diet.

In another twist, eating healthy fats—the types that support the heart, like the omega-3s in tuna and the monounsaturated fat in olive oil—does not seem to cause weight gain. A trial published in *The Lancet Diabetes & Endocrinology* showed that people who followed a Mediterranean diet rich in vegetables and fat for five years lost more weight than those who were told to eat low-fat. A related study found that people who followed a high-fat diet reduced their risk of cardiovascular disease by about 30% compared with those instructed to eat a low-fat diet.

"After hearing for 40 years how eating fat makes you fat and how we have to count calories to control our weight, people are afraid of foods that humans have enjoyed and viewed as healthy for hundreds of years, like olive oil, nuts, avocado, fatty fish, even dark chocolate," says Ludwig. "These foods are among the most healthful foods in existence, even though they are loaded with calories."

Real, natural foods with fiber, protein and fat are so satisfying that you'll naturally eat less of them, the new thinking goes. "If the meal contains all three, then the food will move more slowly through the GI [gastrointestinal] tract," says Mira Ilic, a clinical dietitian at the Cleveland Clinic. When a food takes its time passing through the body, you feel fuller longer. And that helps you naturally regulate your calorie intake.

Instead of choosing a meal based on calories, Ilic advises picking foods from all three categories: one high in fiber, like a vegetable or whole grain; a protein source (think chicken or salmon); and a healthy fat, like a salad with olive oil and chopped avocado.

But it's still possible to overdo it, even on healthy foods. The biggest temptations are typically peanut butter and almond butter, which are often eaten by the spoonful, says Ilic. She likes the "healthy plate" method of foolproof portion control: assembling half a plate of nonstarchy vegetables; a quarter plate of protein; and a quarter plate of quality carbs, like whole grains or legumes. Foods with healthy fats may also pop up in the protein and carb parts of the plate, and if you stick to that formula, you'll be

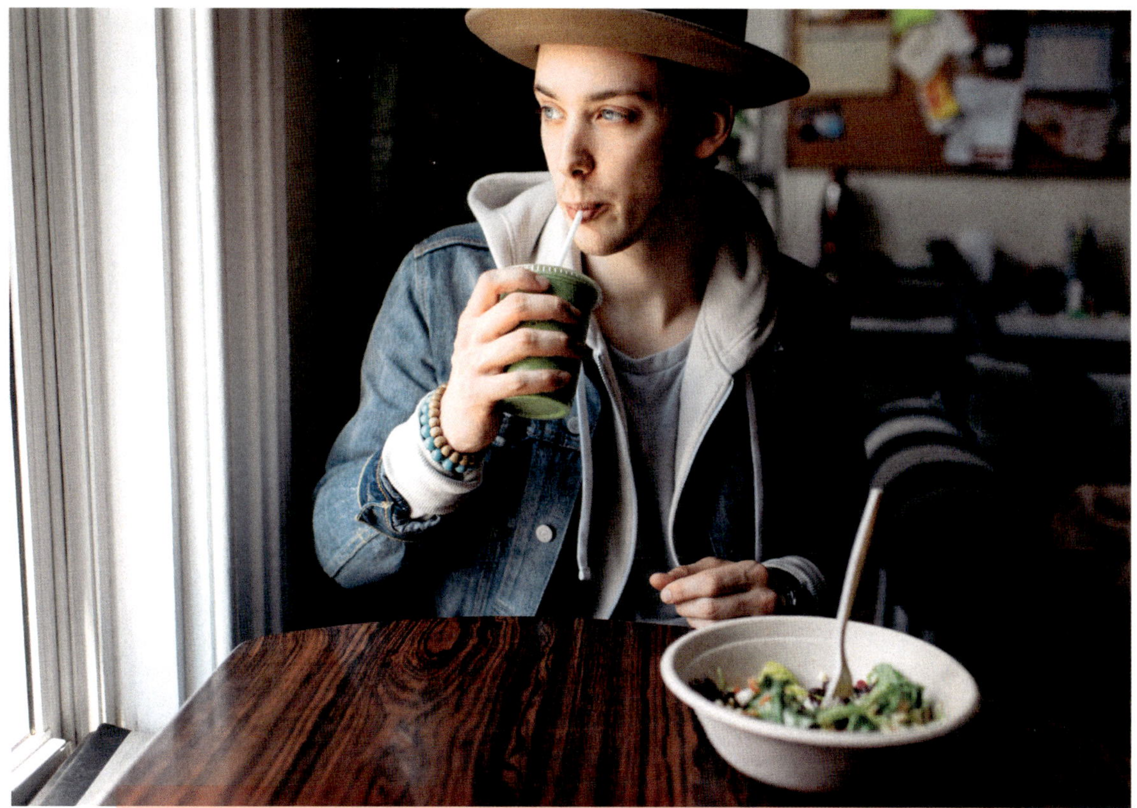

By eating balanced, veggie-rich meals that include protein and healthy fat, you help your body regulate blood sugar and weight.

less likely to overeat them. After creating so well-rounded a meal, you'll find it easier to keep the amount of good fat you add to it in check.

Another way to guard against overeating healthy-but-rich foods is to slow down at the table. "A lot of people are eating way too fast," says Ilic. "It takes a minimum of 20 minutes for the brain to pick up on satiety, the fullness of the stomach, and you miss the cue of being full if you're eating too quickly."

Tune in to your hunger

Recent research found that when people did a short mindfulness exercise called a body-scan meditation—in which you take stock of how you feel inside—they were better able to pick up on internal cues that signal hunger and fullness. People who are more mindful have also been shown to experience fewer weight fluctuations over time.

Even though eating quality calories will help you crave treats less, there's still room for the occasional indulgence. Ludwig is a fan of dark chocolate, which has heart, brain and satiety benefits. If that doesn't do it for you, you can keep the occasional cookie in the mix. "After cleaning the metabolic slate and lowering their insulin, people may be able to enjoy pastries, pasta, etc., in moderation," says Ludwig. If you miss these foods, he recommends experimenting to see what you can handle before cravings are triggered. "For others whose metabolism doesn't tolerate that as much, the benefits of being in control of hunger and not having to fight cravings will be much greater than the fleeting pleasures of those processed carbohydrates."

As for Rabe, she ended her year of dodging calories by embarking on a new one in which she embraced fat and reduced sugar. She lost about as much weight while gaining leanness, strength and a steadier stream of energy. "I feel so much freer to not be restricted and obsessed over calories," she says. "I've made some really major changes in the quality of my diet, and I feel I can sustain them."

Best of all, ditching the meal math renewed her love for food, so much so that she started her own cooking blog.

Rabe says she'll never go back to counting calories. "I'm internally motivated to eat the way I do, because I enjoy it," she says. "I like the way I feel now." □

Raising Kids Who Are Body Positive

I wanted my daughter to have a healthy body image and a healthy relationship with food. My first step: to stop nitpicking my own shape

> ***By Jancee Dunn***

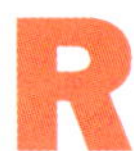

RECENTLY I WAS FRETTING AS I TRIED ON A DRESS FOR a big work event. I stood in front of the mirror, turning this way and that, wondering if it made me look too pear-shaped.

My 9-year-old daughter joined me as I assessed my reflection. "You have such a nice, round hiney," she said, giving it a pat.

I quickly shifted my morose expression into neutral and told her she was right. "I do have a nice, round hiney," I pronounced, and grabbed my bag. Yes, my response was slightly stilted. But I've become acutely aware of the power my words have when I talk about my body in front of my kid.

That means no diet talk. No comments about another person's weight. No complimenting my kid at the expense of myself ("You're gorgeous, but yeesh, look at my stomach rolls!"). And no moaning about how guilty I feel after I've had too much guacamole.

The language that we use when we speak about food is especially important, says New York psychotherapist Claudia Glaser-Mussen. Parents, she says, should avoid absolutes. "When you say, 'Oh, I was so bad, I ate that extra piece of pie,' it teaches kids that food is binary and to be seen as good/bad," she says. By extension, a kid could think that *they* are good or bad. This, says Glaser-Mussen, attaches shame to eating and makes it harder to get back to base-

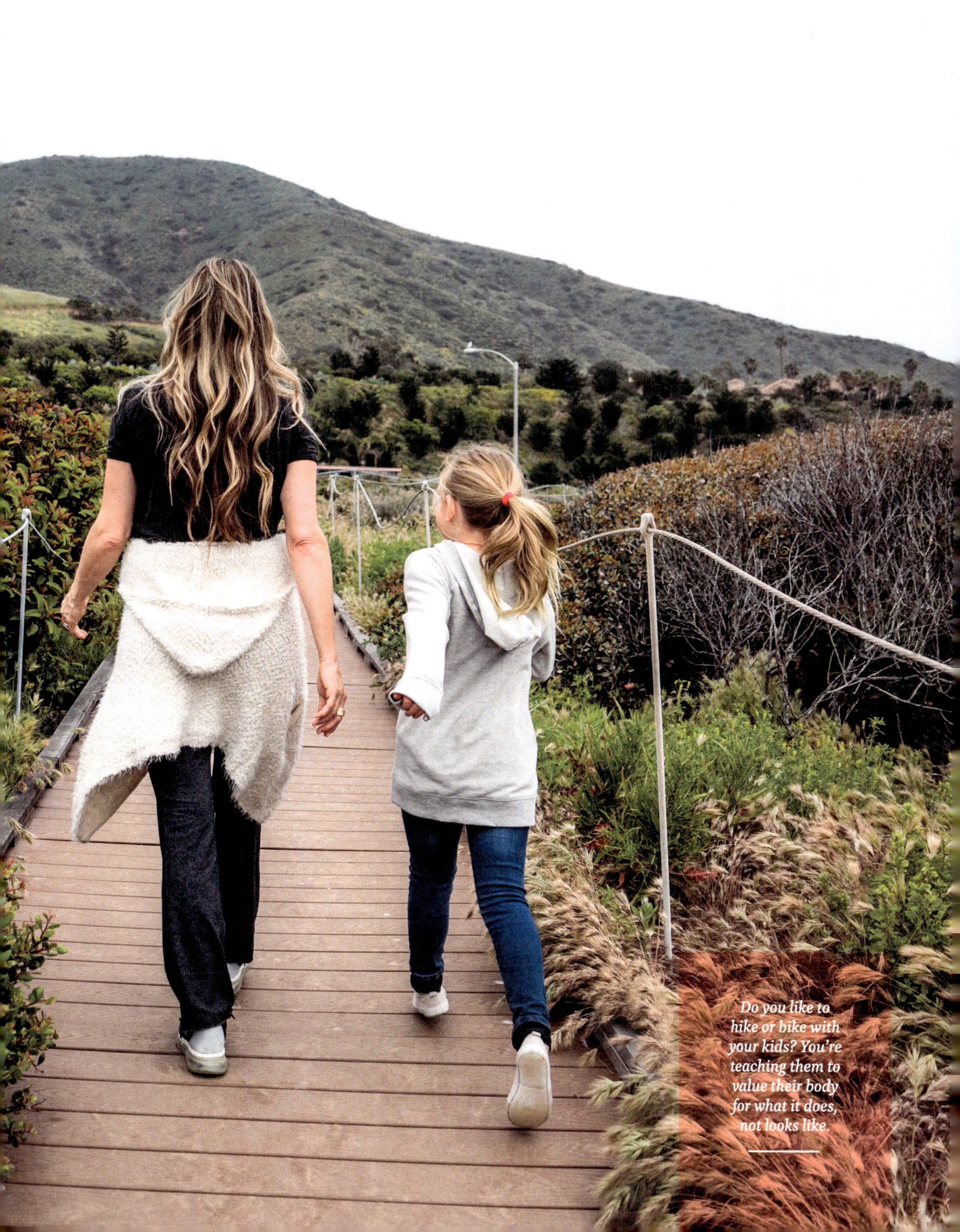

Do you like to hike or bike with your kids? You're teaching them to value their body for what it does, not looks like.

line when you indulge on something less-than-ideal.

I started paying more attention to the way I talked about eating after I had a conversation with Alan Kazdin, director of the Yale Parenting Center. He told me that kids learn behaviors by watching and listening to their parents—what psychologists call modeling. Like some sort of high-level security camera, kids are observing you all the time, whether you're aware of it or not.

And it goes much deeper than just mimicking what you say and do. Kazdin told me that research has demonstrated that there are special cells in the brain called mirror neurons. If I pick up a banana to eat and my daughter is watching me, her brain fires cells that are the equivalent of her hand picking up the banana as well. This suggests, Kazdin said, that seeing a behavior forges the same neural connections that you make from practicing the behavior. In other words, modeling can actually change the brain.

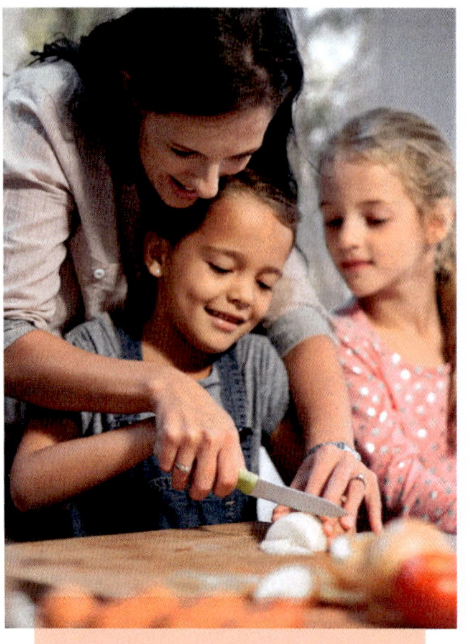

Kids who cook are more likely to choose healthy foods.

"Modeling is so important," Kazdin told me. "I think it's nice in some ways that parents don't really realize the responsibilities that they have and that their behavior is being observed all the time," he said. "It's really daunting."

But I had never entirely realized how thoroughly children absorb their mothers' negative body talk, or NBT—and how early their feelings about their body image take root. A 2015 report from Common Sense Media found that girls as young as 5 who think their moms are dissatisfied with their bodies are more likely to be unhappy with their own. Even more disheartening was a 2010 report that found that nearly a third of kids ages 5 to 6 choose an ideal body size that's thinner than their own perceived size.

Nor are boys immune. A 2012 study published in the journal *Pediatrics* found that two thirds of middle school and high school boys exercised regularly not to improve their health but to be more toned. A 2016 University of Chicago study found that eating disorders tend to begin at an earlier age with boys—at age 13, rather than age 14 for girls.

I noticed that I was practicing NBT all the time. We do it as a way to give a compliment to a friend ("I wish I had your thighs; mine are huge!"). We do it to assure others that we don't think we're better than anyone else. We do it to make each other laugh. In a recent group text with friends, one volunteered that when she looks down at her smartphone—the worst angle imaginable—her resulting double chin made her look like Walter Matthau. We all chimed in with our own comparisons, heavy on America's forefathers—Ben Franklin, John Quincy Adams.

It can be reassuring that other people have the same thoughts as you do—and indeed, experts think this body bashing evolved as a way for women to bond with friends by showing vulnerability. Unfortunately, research shows that airing insecurities with friends actually makes you feel worse.

Not only that, but like some sort of pernicious virus, this behavior is catching. A 2012 report in the journal *Psychology of Women Quarterly* shows that engaging in Negative Body Talk prompts other women to do it too. NBT is not harmless chitchat; it has long-term consequences. A 2015 study published in the journal *Adolescent Health, Medicine and Therapeutics* found that the frequency with which teen girls and boys participate in "fat talk" is correlated with eating-disordered behavior.

And the more we do it, the more it becomes the norm—making it harder for those with healthy attitudes toward their bodies to speak up.

But of course, it's hard to stop NBT from bubbling up in your brain. When I was recently in a dressing room, trying on clothes—without my daughter—I was cursing at my nice, round hiney as I tried to stuff it into a pair of jeans.

And I am constantly fighting food-related guilt.

I have an addiction to crunchy cheese puffs (they're "natural," and I buy them from my health-food store, but who am I kidding?). I have been known to mindlessly polish off a four-serving bag until the only thing that remains is a crusty coating of orange-colored dust on my fingers. Afterward, I slide into a pit of guilt (which, by the way, is pretty much the worst motivator ever).

But I try my hardest to keep those thoughts to myself. I want my daughter's feelings around food to be different than mine were when I was growing up in the '80s. My mom, a former Southern beauty queen, tried every diet under the sun to maintain her "figure": the Grapefruit Diet, the Liquid Diet. In our family, food was often something to subdue, to avoid, to fear. She zealously measured portions. She lived on gallons of peach-flavored iced tea. A "special treat" was one SnackWell cookie. And exercise was not a fun activity but grim punishment for overindulging.

So with my own daughter, I focus on how food makes you feel rather than how it makes you look. I try to make exercise a fun part of life, rather than penance for too much Mexican food. Sylvie and I take long walks together, or we kick around a soccer ball in the park.

I take her with me when I go grocery shopping too. I've taught her how to read food labels, and nothing gives her more pleasure than to run over with a can of soda, gravely announcing, with wide eyes, that it contains 40 grams of sugar. (Kids love to be sanctimonious.)

Although I do wonder sometimes if this zeal might tip into being overly focused on food. It's a fine line to walk. I tell my kid to avoid foods with ingredients you can't pronounce, but childhood is full of them: supermarket sheet cakes at kids' parties, fast food on family road trips. I try to be easygoing about it all. We call those things "sometime" foods (rather than "always" foods, like spinach).

Most things are not "nevers." A few weeks ago, I took my daughter and one of her friends to a diner, and she ordered Jell-O for dessert. When I asked the boy if he wanted some too, he shook his head. "My mom says that stuff is poison," he said. Jeez. OK, it's a color not found in nature. And maybe a flavor, too. But poison?

Girls as young as 5 who think their moms are unhappy with their bodies are more likely to be unhappy with their own.

And I try to make sure that at least a few times a week, we put on some music and cook dinner together. Cooking is, of course, a vital life skill, but according to some experts, it's the single most important thing you can do for your health. Research shows that having kids join in on cooking meals is one of the best ways to get them motivated to eat more whole foods. (When you're whipping up something at home, you're generally not throwing in corn syrup or sodium benzoate.) A 2014 study of kids ages 5 through 12 from the Centers for Disease Control and Prevention found that getting kids involved in the kitchen made them more likely to choose healthy foods.

What's key to modeling a healthy relationship with food, says Glaser-Mussen, is to practice mindful eating as a family. "Research has shown that highlighting pleasure around food and appreciating all food naturally slows down eating."

If I happen to do the opposite and huff down multiple slices of pizza—it's pretty much impossible for me to slow down around it—I make sure that afterward, Sylvie doesn't see me do a shame spiral. Tone is key, so I'll laugh and say something like, "Whoa, I didn't need that last piece. But it was good! Eh, I'll eat healthier tomorrow."

To that end, I have dessert almost every night—not a banana split, necessarily, but an ice cream cone or a cookie (or two). I try to have desserts loud and proud, to get across that sweets are not something to fear or obsess over.

I've benefited from the modeling behavior. One of the beauties of becoming a parent is that it can be a do-over—an opportunity to act the way you wish you had in the first place. When I first started making body-positive pronouncements like "I'm so glad my body is strong," I felt like a dopey cartoon puppet.

It's easy to correct your words but much harder to silence your hectoring internal critic. Our attitudes about food and weight are pretty deeply ingrained. But here's the thing: over time, some of my sunny statements that I've made for my kid's benefit have not entirely been lip service.

Sometimes—just sometimes—I actually believe what I say. □

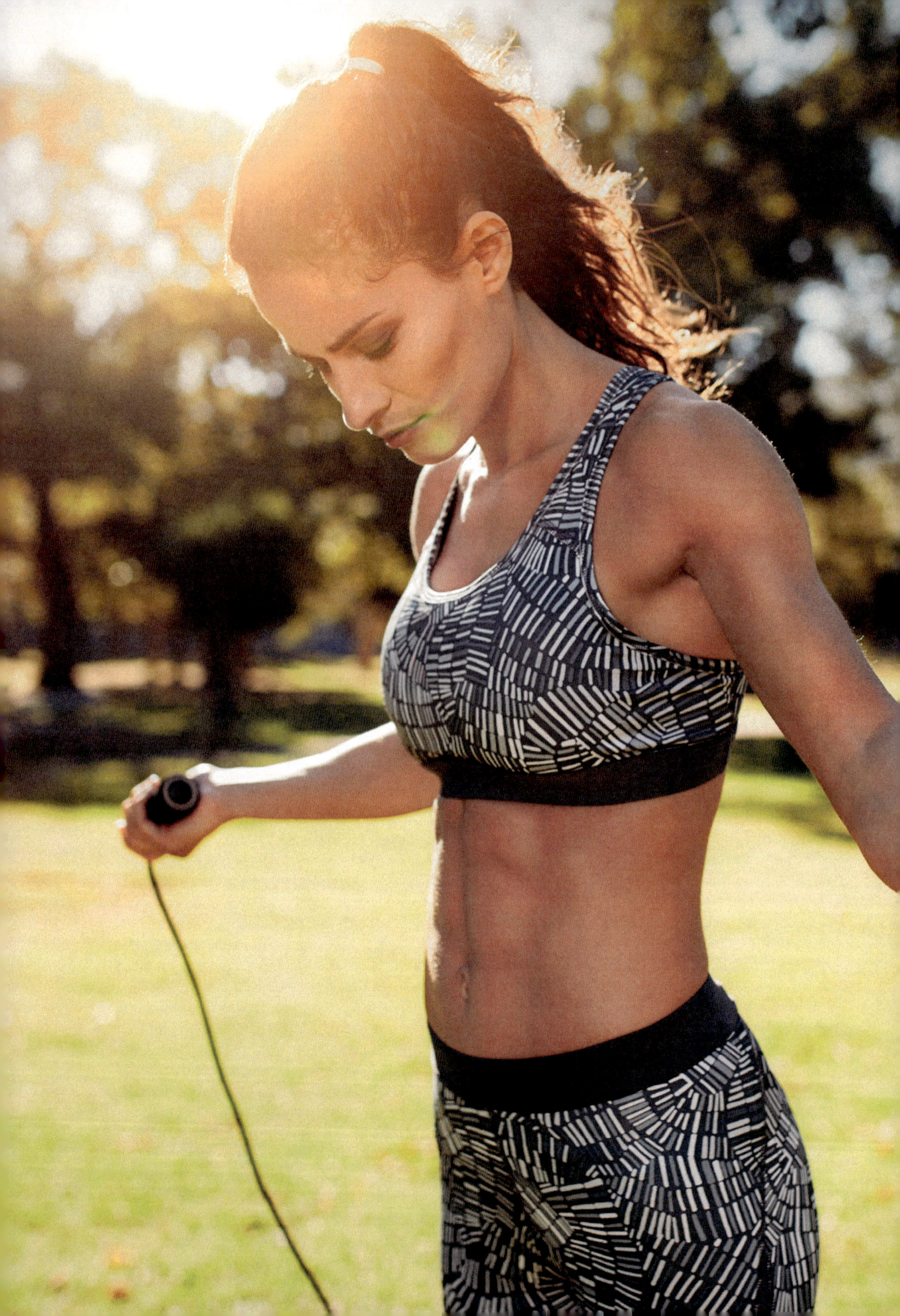

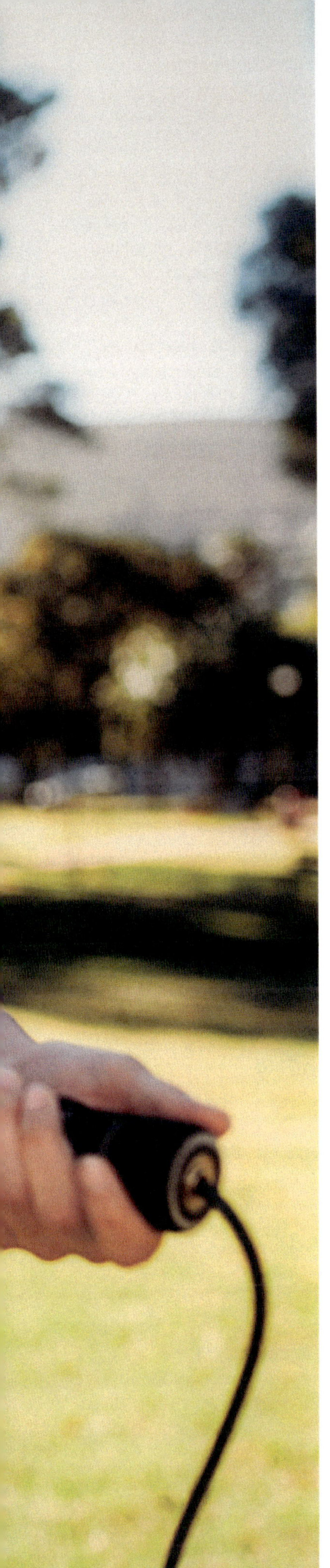

The Definitive Guide to Body Fat

Some good fat can improve our metabolism. Another type can wrap around the heart. Discover how body fat can help and harm our health

› **By Hallie Levine**

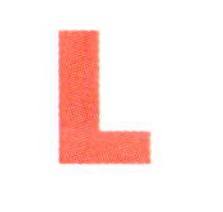

ET'S FACE IT: FAT HAS GOTTEN AN UNFORTUNATE rap. We curse the dimpled cellulite that has settled on our thighs and survey the pudge around our belly with a quick poke and a disapproving eye. But here's the thing: Fat isn't just a place where your body dumps extra calories. It's an organ that can help, or harm, your health. (One type, brown fat, can actually turn your body into a calorie-burning machine!) "Everyone has fat, even Olympic marathon runners," says Osama Hamdy, medical director of the Obesity Clinical Program at Harvard University's Joslin Diabetes Center. "Simply put, we need it to survive." The trick is understanding the differences between the kinds of fat and keeping them in balance with diet, exercise and some common sense.

About subcutaneous fat

Where it is: Directly underneath your skin. Subcutaneous fat can be anywhere: not just in your belly and butt but also your arms, legs, even your face.
What it does: In addition to storing energy and pro-

viding essential padding for your body, it has another important job: it generates the hormone adiponectin, which helps regulate insulin production. "Paradoxically, the fatter you are, the less adiponectin you produce, which means that your body has trouble regulating insulin, increasing the risk of heart disease and diabetes," Hamdy says.

How to get rid of it: Cutting calories is crucial for overall weight loss, but getting moving counts too: women who walked, cycled or took public transportation to work had about 1.5% less body fat than those who drove, according to a U.K. study. "It's proof that those little bursts of activity count when it comes to burning fat," notes Pamela Peeke, the author of *Body for Life for Women*. "Even just walking from the train station or bus to your office can burn on average an extra hundred calories."

Already active? Ramp it up. "When you take your workout up a notch, you reach VO2 max—that's the level of exertion where you have the optimal breakdown of body fat," Peeke explains. "It also fools your body into thinking that you're working out minutes after you've stopped, so you're still burning calories."

Visceral fat

Where it is: Nestled deep within your belly, where it pads the spaces around your abdominal organs. You can't feel or grab it.

What it does: Visceral fat has been dubbed "toxic" fat, and for good reason: "It secretes inflammatory proteins called cytokines that affect insulin production and increase inflammation throughout the body, which raises the risk of developing Type 2 diabetes and heart disease," Hamdy says. You can't directly measure visceral fat unless you undergo an MRI or a CT scan.

The next best thing? Grab a tape measure and wind it around your waist; if your midsection is more than 35 inches, you most likely have too much visceral fat, Hamdy says. A Mayo Clinic study published in 2014 found that Caucasian women with waist sizes above 37 inches were more likely to die from heart or respiratory disease.

Another sign of trouble appears when your numbers are off, meaning you've got low HDL (good) cholesterol and elevated blood glucose and triglyceride levels. "When a woman who has been lean most of her life gains 10 to 20 pounds at age 40 or so, she may not even be technically overweight, but it's usually visceral fat that's adding the extra weight," explains Caroline Cederquist, a bariatric physician in Naples, Fla., and the author of *The MD Factor Diet*.

How to blast it off: "To mobilize visceral fat, a balanced diet is essential," Cederquist says. "Eat lean protein throughout the day while controlling your carb and fat intake." For keeping visceral fat off, cardio is the way to go: a 2011 Duke University study found that regular aerobic exercise, the equivalent of jogging about 12 miles a week at 80% maximum heart rate, was the best workout for losing visceral fat in particular.

Brown fat (a.k.a. good fat)

Where it is: Mainly around your neck, collarbone and chest. For years, researchers assumed that it was present primarily in infants, helping to keep them warm, and that it gradually disappeared during childhood. But in 2009, studies revealed that some adults still have brown cells.

What it does: This buzzed-about "good" fat becomes metabolically active when we're exposed to cold temperatures, burning up energy. "Since brown fat is used to generate heat, it burns more calories at rest," says Ruth Loos, professor of preventive medicine at Mount Sinai Hospital in New York City. Fifty grams (about 4 tablespoons) of brown fat, if maximally stimulated, could torch about 300 calories a day.

How to beef it up: Since brown fat is activated by cold, prepare to shiver. According to a study in *Cell Metabolism*, folks who spent 10 to 15 minutes in temperatures below 60 degrees produced a hormone called irisin, which appears to make white fat cells act like brown fat; they got a similar boost from an hour of moderate exercise at warmer temperatures. And keep your thermostat low: an Australian study showed that men who lived in homes set to 66 degrees generated 40% more brown fat than when they lived in higher temperatures.

About body-fat percentage

The best way to determine whether you're carrying too much flab is to check your body-fat percentage. A healthy range is between 20% and 25% for young women and up to 30% after age 50, Peeke says. Skip the skin calipers (they pinch the skin around your

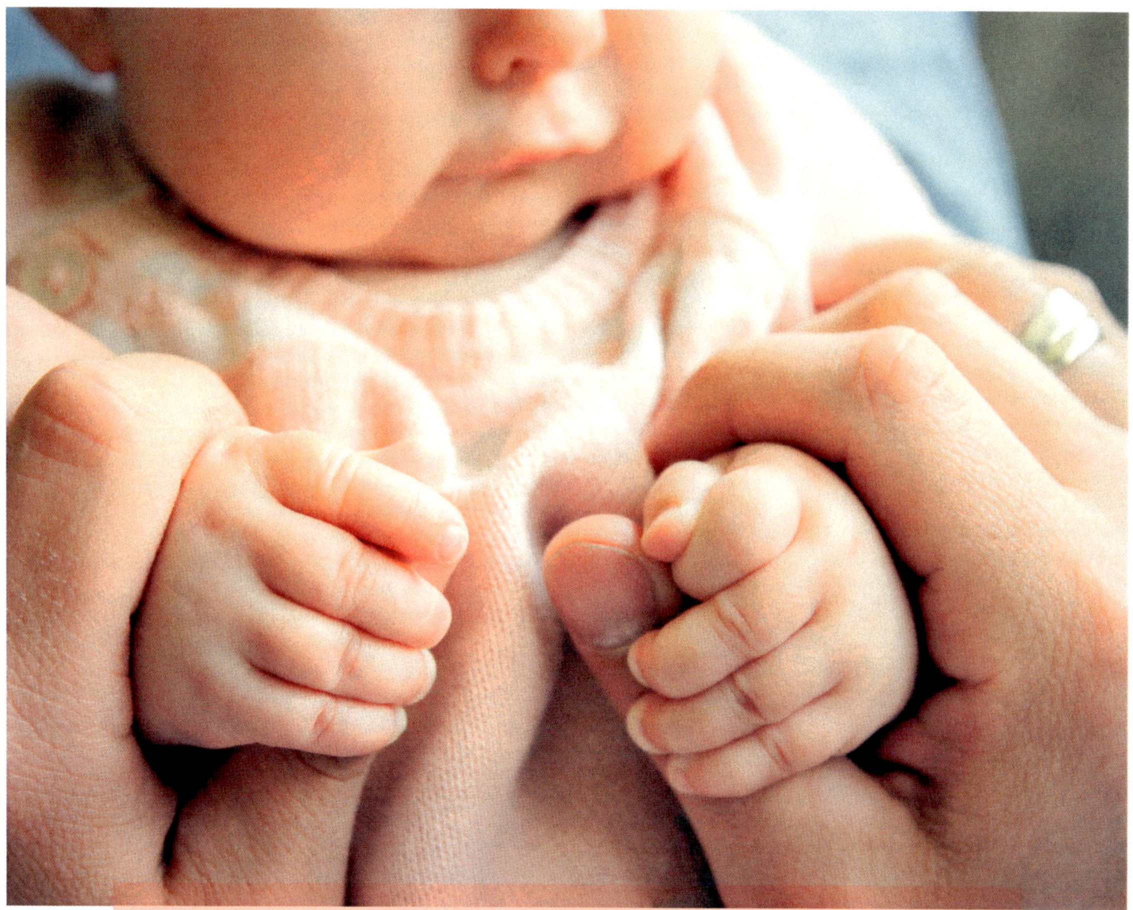

Healthy rolls: a baby is born with brown-fat cells, which burn energy to help keep the baby warm.

upper arm, thigh and stomach); results can be off by as much as 5%. Peeke's recommendation: an at-home bioelectrical impedance scale, which sends an electrical current through your body and measures how fast it returns. Other methods, such as underwater weighing (you're dunked into a pool to measure your body fat) and DEXA scans (which use an x-ray to determine body composition, including body fat, lean muscle and bone density), are more accurate, but you'll have to go to a health clinic to get measured.

Cellulite explained

Skin dimples happen when subcutaneous fat cells collect in pockets and push against the connective tissue under your skin. You can minimize their appearance by staying at a healthy weight and doing strength-training moves (more muscle equals tauter skin). Caffeine-infused creams (such as Clarins Body Lift Cellulite Control) can temporarily de-puff fat cells for a smoother look.

The danger of ectopic fat

Ectopic fat has the same metabolic properties as visceral fat, but instead of padding your abdominal organs, it settles in your heart, liver, pancreas and muscles. "Most of us have only a few pounds of ectopic fat," Hamdy says. "Even so, it's dangerous because it's inside vital organs and can increase the risk of heart disease, liver damage and Type 2 diabetes."

The only way to tell if you have ectopic fat is by getting an MRI or a CT scan. One key way to avoid this problem is to stay active. The more you sit, the more likely you are to have this fat around your heart, according to a University of California, San Diego, study.

How to actually burn off fat

Resistance train: A strength workout that incorporates high-intensity interval training (HIIT) will help burn calories and fat stores at a higher rate than one done in straight sets, says trainer Gunnar Peterson.

The drill: do eight repetitions of different types of body-weight-resistance activities (chin-ups, squats, burpees, etc.), alternating 20 seconds of work with 10 seconds of rest.

Rest: Yet another benefit of getting a good night of sleep: a Brigham Young University study found that women who slept between 8 and 8½ hours a night had the lowest levels of body fat. Why? Lack of sleep can wreak havoc on hormones that control fat metabolism. If you have trouble getting a solid seven or eight hours of rest, try shutting down your devices at least one hour before bedtime. Also make sure your room is dark; light from alarm clocks and the street can interrupt sleep.

Relax: Doing yoga can reduce cortisol levels—high levels of the stress hormone have been linked to belly fat. In fact, obese postmenopausal women who practiced yoga for 16 weeks reported significant reductions in visceral fat, according to a Korean study.

If you have trouble getting seven or eight hours of rest, try shutting down your devices at least one hour before bedtime.

How age factors in

Childhood: The number of fat cells you have is set early on, so you don't actually get more of them when you gain weight. Instead, those fat cells swell as triglycerides (i.e., fatty acids) are stored in them. If enough fat cells expand in size, your body begins to, well, expand too. Boys tend to be born with more fat cells in their belly, while girls are born with more fat cells in their hips, thighs and butt, in preparation for storing fat during pregnancy.

Adolescence: Between the ages of 9 and 19, the volume of fat in girls more than doubles, due in part to a surge of the female hormone estrogen. "Your body starts producing estrogen in preparation for having a baby and nursing years down the road. That estrogen helps fuel the growth of fat cells," Peeke says.

Post-pregnancy: There's a reason it is so difficult to shed that extra fat after having a baby. It's a throwback to our caveperson days, says Peeke. "It's reserve storage for the demands of breastfeeding," she explains. This helps ensure that new mothers can feed their babies in times of famine. So even though breastfeeding burns about 500 calories a day, your body is hardwired to hold on to some fat deposits, and you may not lose those last 5 or 10 pounds until after you wean.

Menopause: Until this point, most women still store fat around their lower half, but once they go through menopause, their fat-storage patterns mimic men's, which means women may start sporting what looks like a beer belly.

Can you be heavy and healthy?

Some research suggests yes, but the answer isn't entirely clear yet. A 2013 study found that although overweight people may have a higher life expectancy than normal-weight people, they spend those years in poorer health.

"While certain types of fat, particularly subcutaneous fat, may not have the impact on your heart that visceral fat does, they can affect your quality of life," Peeke says. "If you're heavy, you're more likely to develop osteoarthritis or just have trouble moving around."

The best fat-fighting foods

Dairy: People who consumed more dairy while on a low-calorie diet lost 2½ more pounds of fat than those who didn't, according to a review published in the *International Journal of Obesity*.

Proteins: Research has shown that people lose more visceral fat on a lower-carb, higher-protein diet than they do on a low-fat diet that's high in carbohydrates, Hamdy points out.

Oatmeal: For every 10-gram increase in soluble fiber consumed per day, visceral fat was reduced by 3.7% over five years, according to a study at Wake Forest University in Winston-Salem, N.C.

Vegetable oil: Swedish research found that polyunsaturated fats (including omega-6-rich oils such as safflower, soybean and corn) may help prevent you from gaining visceral fat and may even help you build muscle.

Fatty fish: Omega-3s (found in salmon, tuna, mackerel and sardines, as well as flaxseed and walnuts) may help reduce abdominal fat. And—bonus!—they may be protective for your heart too. □

8 WAYS FAT AFFECTS THE FEMALE BODY

Having excess fat—or too little of it—can wreak havoc with a woman's system **BY HALLIE LEVINE**

1: Head » The risk of migraines increases by almost 40% in younger women with general or belly obesity, according to the American Headache Society.

2: Brain » Being underweight was associated with a 36% higher risk of developing dementia, while being obese conferred a 42% higher risk, per a study done at the Johns Hopkins Bloomberg School of Public Health in Baltimore.

3: Heart » One study found that overweight people have a 32% higher risk of coronary artery disease than those at a normal weight.

4: Breasts » After menopause, women who are overweight have a 30% to 60% higher breast-cancer risk than those at a normal weight.

5: Blood sugar » According to a Canadian study, women who had BMIs higher than 30 had a twelvefold higher risk of developing Type 2 diabetes.

6: Ovaries » Six percent of infertility cases are due to being overweight, and 6% are due to being underweight, according to the American Society of Reproductive Medicine.

7: Bones » A Japanese study found that postmenopausal overweight women had a higher risk of getting vertebral fractures; very skinny women were more likely to suffer fractures in the neck and long bones (such as the shin, thigh or forearm).

8: Knees » A U.K. study found that overweight women had six times the risk of developing knee osteoarthritis of their lean counterparts.

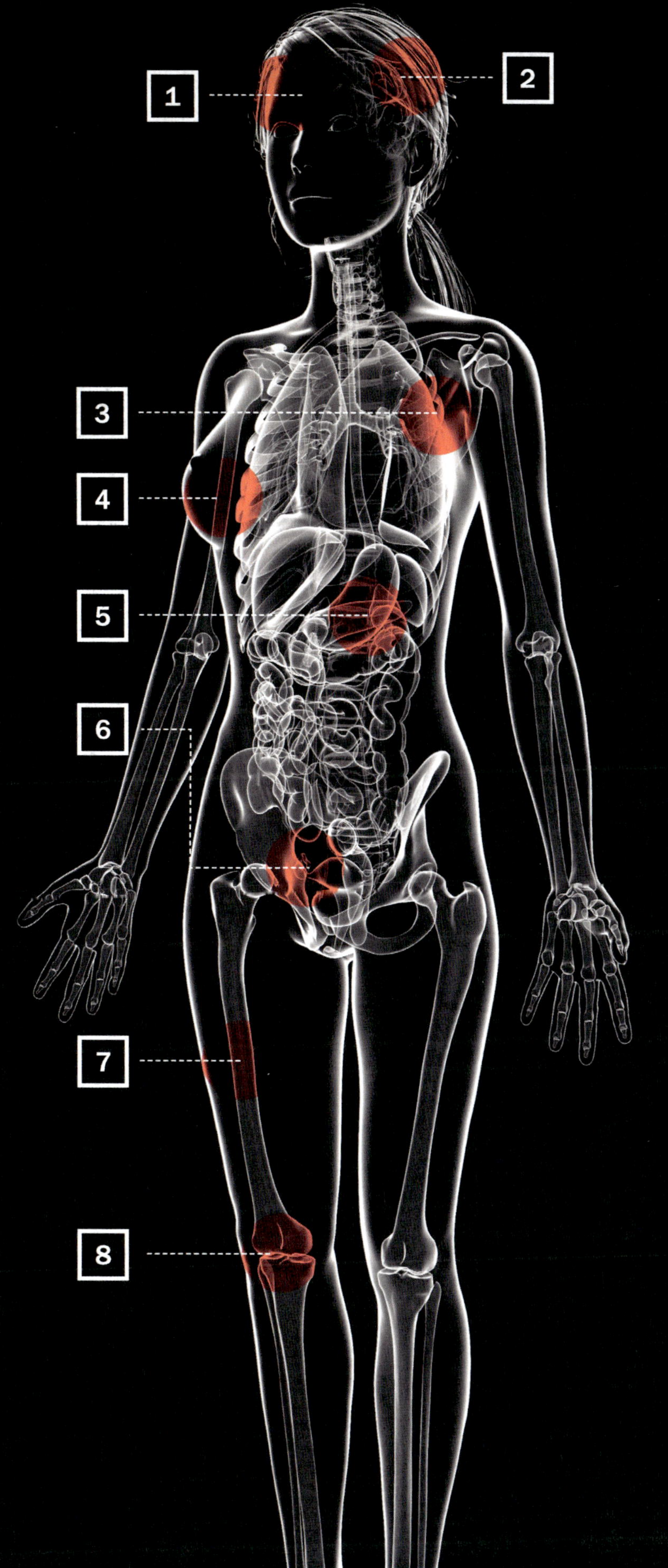

Chapter 2

Clean LIV

How to prevent busy-life gain, tune in to cravings,

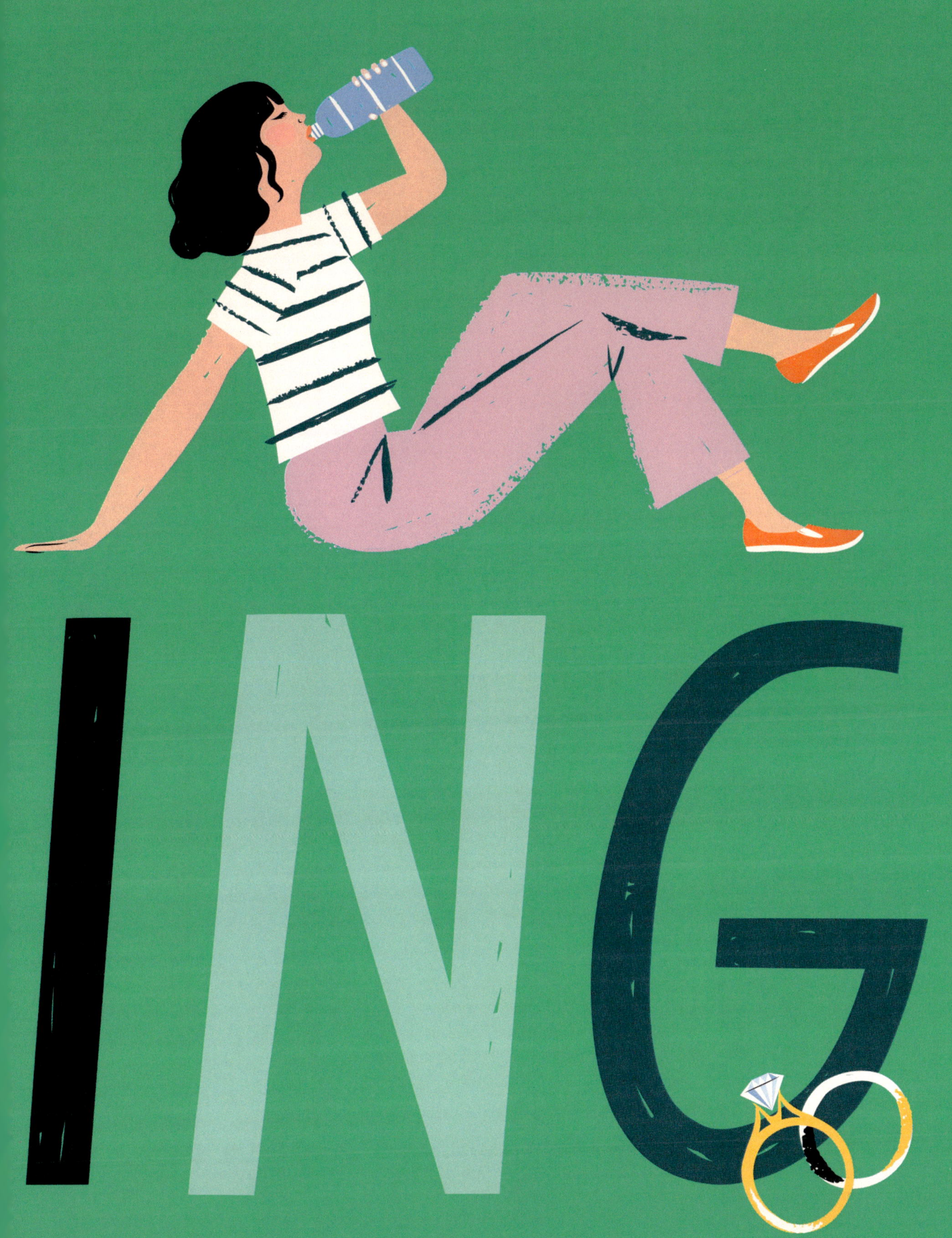

eat well when you're out and find filling whole foods

How Stress Makes Us Gain

What to do when evolution is working against you. Hint: being aware helps

By Kate Rope

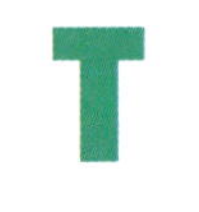

TIM CHAMBERS WAS JUST SHY OF 300 POUNDS WHEN a heart attack scare sent him to the ER. The 51-year-old web developer from Bethesda, Md., had been putting on pounds ever since he entered the working world and held a series of sedentary jobs at internet and computer-game companies. Sitting in the hospital—after fainting on the commuter train while heading home from work—was a "wake-up call" for Chambers, who had had limited success losing weight in the past. "I lost 30 to 40 pounds three or four times in a row," says Chambers. "But then work would become stressful again, and the weight would come back, usually higher."

Stories such as Chambers's are familiar to Rachel Goldman, a Manhattan psychologist who specializes in weight management and stress reduction. When we are under stress, "our health behaviors are the first thing to go," says Goldman. "We say, 'I don't have time to make it to the gym. I don't have time to make healthy food.' " Our overscheduled, fast-paced lives often win out over our best intentions.

But research has uncovered a much deeper interaction, one that goes back to our oldest ancestors and shows how the very system designed to help them survive could be threatening our own health. For years, studies have shown a connection between high levels of the stress hormone cortisol in saliva, urine or blood and being overweight, but a study published in 2017 presented some of the most

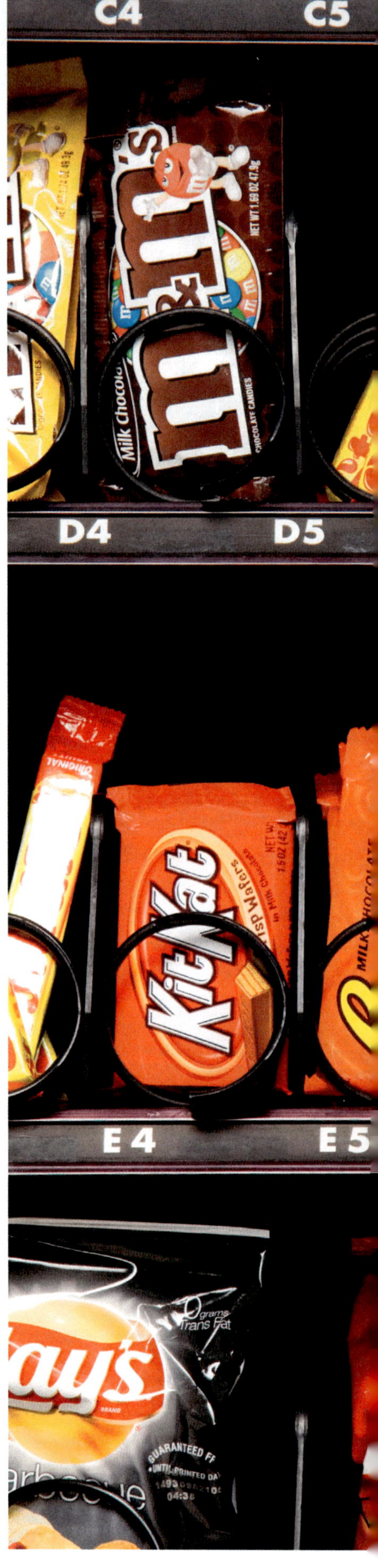

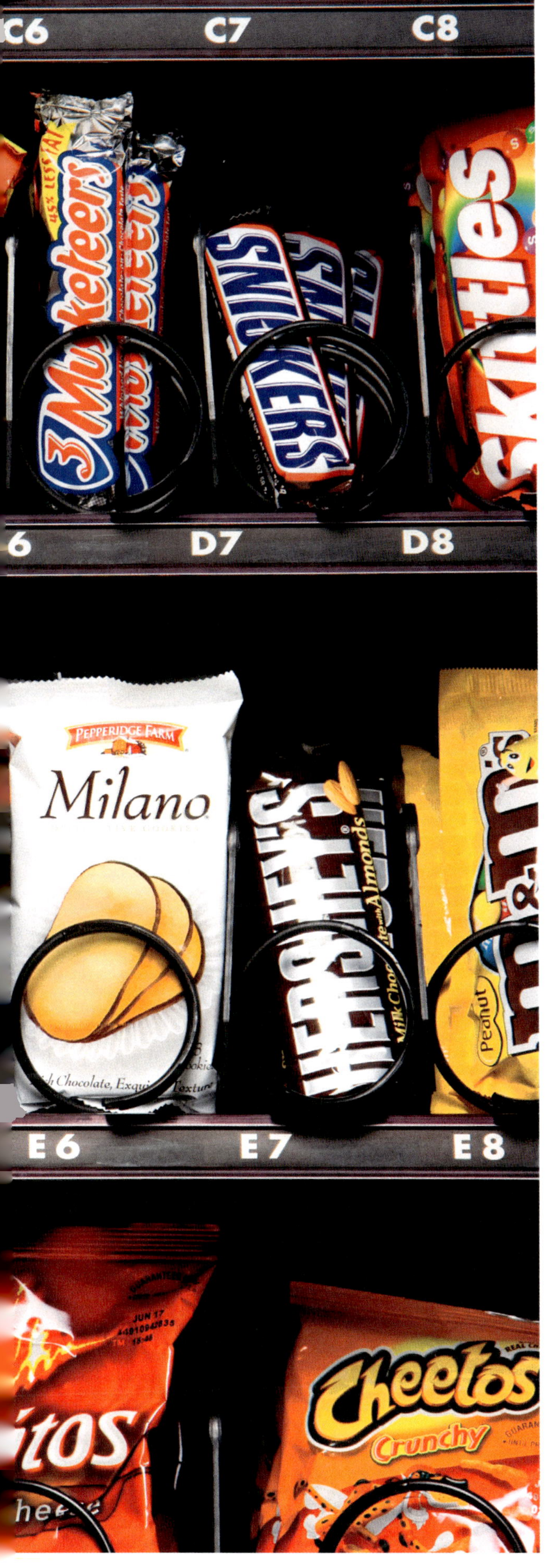

compelling evidence that long-term stress is connected to being overweight. Sarah Jackson, a senior research associate in the department of behavioral science and health at the University College London, measured cortisol levels in hair. "By using hair samples to measure cortisol, we were able to get a better sense of average cortisol levels over a prolonged period," says Jackson. Her research showed "a link between longer-term stress and weight, body mass index, waist circumference and abdominal obesity," says Jackson. "Exposure to this hormone is associated with greater body fatness."

Discovering how cortisol influences weight gain—and attempting to interrupt that process—is another important area of research and the life's work of Pamela Peeke, an assistant professor of medicine at the University of Maryland School of Medicine, a Pew Foundation Scholar in nutrition and metabolism and the author of *The Hunger Fix*. It all comes back to the fight-or-flight response.

Evolution designed our bodies to produce instant energy when we are under threat. Our bodies break down both fat and glucose from the liver to use as fuel and circulate it throughout the body "so that you've got everything you need to run or beat the hell out of a predator," says Peeke. At the same time, our body is depositing fat in the safest place possible to have energy later—under our abdominal muscles. "It's the most precious fat depot in the human body, and your body wants to protect it for survival," she explains. After a fight for your life is over, your body is primed to replenish the calories lost during it, and "you get a cortisol-stimulated appetite to be able to replete the calories your body assumes you've expended," explains Peeke.

It's all a "beautiful response," she adds. For a caveperson, that is. This system keeps them safe from danger and helps them enjoy berries after a long run away from a predator without gaining weight. For a modern-day desk jockey, the system is less helpful. Stress like mounting deadlines and climbing interest rates leave us revved up and fist deep in the office candy bowl. And it becomes a vicious cycle: your body stores more fat deep in your tissues—where it likes to stay put—and you end up eating more.

"What you have is fabulous primal software that is being used inappropriately in today's 21st-century world," says Peeke. "And we have so many metabolic consequences from that dysfunction, including the No. 1 disordered eating pattern—binge eating."

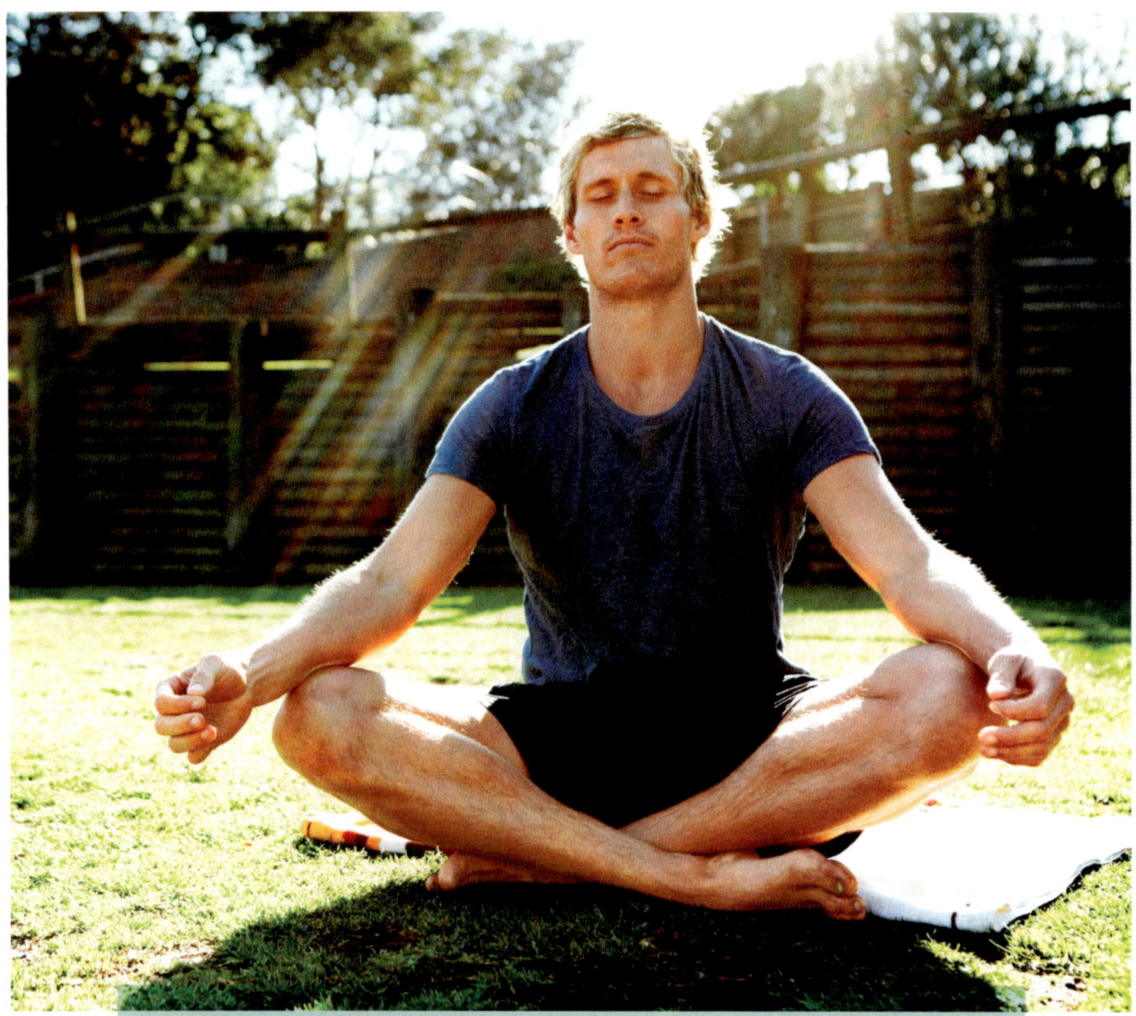

Why meditate? When you have a daily coping ritual, you bring your stress level back to baseline, so it doesn't spill over and start to harm your body.

What's more, rather than living a life punctuated by the threat of a saber-toothed tiger, many of us live a life of lesser but continuous stresses. It's something our bodies were not designed to handle. "When our body never gets out of that fight-or-flight mode, it becomes chronic stress," says Goldman.

You may not realize the impact stress is having on you. "Most people are walking around with ridiculously high levels of stress hormones and don't even know it," says Peeke. And our body's primal reward system pushes us toward one of two things to soothe itself: sex or food. Sex is scarce in our modern workaday world, but vending machines? Plentiful.

And here's why we call the high-fat, high-calorie foods in them "comfort foods." When we eat them, our cortisol levels decrease and we feel a sense of relief. In fact, says Peeke, "people who overeat under stress actually feel a drug-related anesthesia." That sounds—and probably feels—pretty good. The problem is that it is short-lived, she adds: "You just ate a load of sugar, your insulin levels skyrocketed, and now you have all of these metabolic consequences."

This kind of stress eating, which anyone can fall prey to, might lead to your typical middle-age weight gain of 20 to 30 pounds. But genetics and life experiences can turn stress eating into addictive eating, with much more serious weight and health consequences. There are many genes—ones related to addiction, metabolism, diabetes, depression and anxiety—that factor into a propensity to overeat or gain weight. When they interact with negative experiences in childhood, the effect can be exponential. According to research from the Harvard Nurses' Health Study, children who experience the chronic stress of abuse—verbal or physical—or have other traumatic incidents in their childhood are more likely to end up overweight or obese. Early on, says Peeke, they have few outlets to manage their stress, so they often turn to food, developing a brain-body feedback loop that can actually alter their genes' messaging to predispose them to addictive eating.

In fact, the first study to examine the connection between child abuse and food addiction, published in the journal *Obesity* in 2013, found that for women, a history of any kind of abuse led to a 90% increase in the risk of developing a food addiction.

But lesser events can also put you at risk for stress-related weight gain. "Stress is in the eyes of the beholder," says Peeke. "The guy sitting at the desk with all those deadlines? In his brain, he is under ridiculous strain. You don't need a building to fall on your head to develop addictive-like eating behaviors—they fall on a spectrum."

Children who grow up with the chronic stress of abuse or other trauma are more likely to end up overweight or obese.

And that spectrum is where Tim Chambers found himself after his health scare. "It is easy when you are stressed out to only worry about getting through that day," says Chambers. "It's very easy to have a short-term mindset."

Sitting in that hospital room, Chambers changed his. He decided to make three lifestyle changes that he could track every day—exercise, sleep and food—to create a "chain" of healthy behavior. "If I would get enough sleep, get 10,000 steps, eat within my allotted calories and go to the gym three or four times a week, that was not breaking the chain," says Chambers. "I would try to go for the longest period I could without breaking it. If I did break it, I would just pick it back up again." In two years, he lost 115 pounds, which he has kept off for two years and counting.

Chambers's three-point plan hits several of the suggestions Goldman gives her clients. "Water intake, food intake, movement, sleep and stress."

To reduce stress, Goldman recommends having at least three adaptive coping mechanisms that you can actually see yourself doing in times of stress—such as cooking, cleaning, deep breathing, calling a friend, taking a walk or taking a bath. "If you are participating in daily coping mechanisms, it's much easier to bring your stress level back to baseline," she says.

For people who have a history of trauma, Peeke recommends finding a therapist—a psychologist or a licensed social worker—who has certifications in trauma-based work. It also helps to equip yourself with techniques that can fill in for that 20-minute run from the woolly mammoth. "One of the best things you can do to calm the storm—bar none—is meditation," says Peeke. "We've done tremendous epigenetic studies, and what we've found is that regular meditators have a decrease in both the level of stress hormone as well as in the expression of inflammatory genes. The result is better control of overeating and weight gain. Literally, you dial it down. How cool is that?"

"Go for meditative walks, meditative runs, bring on yoga. How about tai chi? Do the kinds of physical activity where you have a chance to get lost in it," she adds. "When I'm in the pool doing laps, nobody is bothering me. It is exquisitely meditative." That combo "will be able to reverse so much of what's taking place in both your mind and body."

But it won't happen overnight, shares Chambers. "You have to have a sense that if I go for a really long walk right now or if I go to the gym and work rather than just eat, it will be better for me. What's tough is that it's not instant gratification like eating, but as you get through the things that are stressing you, and you look back, it helps you have more belief in it the next time."

Chambers's faith and patience have helped him create his own brain-to-body feedback loop, this time a positive one. He has kept the weight off, and he reports that while his "external stressors are about the same as they've always been, my management of them has been different than it has been my entire adult life." □

All About Cravings

Rich and sugary foods trigger our innate survival instinct. Can't swear them off? You don't have to, according to the latest science

> **By Sunny Sea Gold**

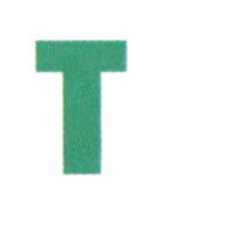

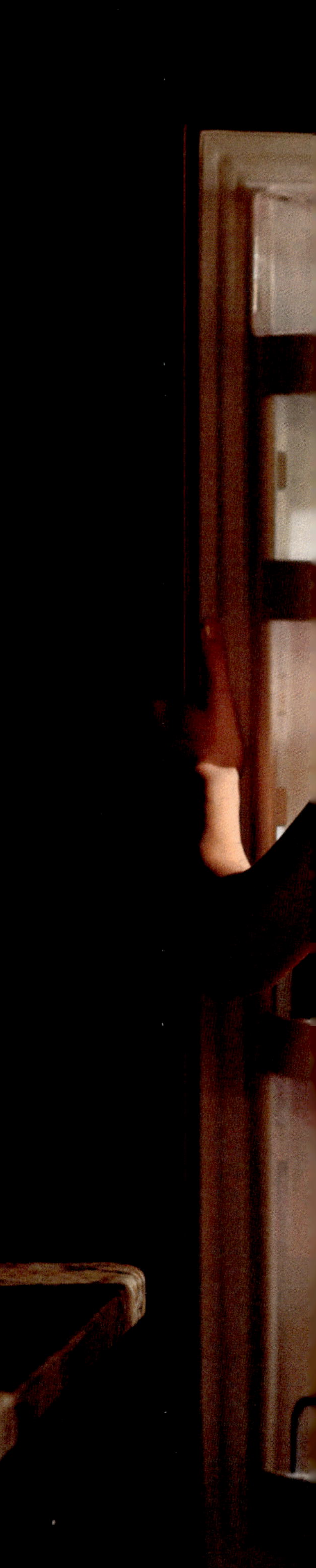

HE FIRST THING YOU NEED TO KNOW ABOUT FOOD cravings? That nearly everything you know about them is wrong. Over the past several decades, well-meaning experts—and, yes, some profit-motivated diet peddlers—have told us cravings are something to be resisted at all costs. "Giving in" is not only harmful to one's health, the story goes, it also shows a distasteful lack of willpower! The reality is quite the contrary, top researchers and dietitians report.

Food cravings are a natural part of humans' strive to survive, says Mark L. Andermann, a neuroscientist who studies hunger and eating behavior at Harvard Medical School. "Your brain is programmed from birth to act as if there won't be enough calories in the world," he explains. Famine stalks countries such as Somalia and Sudan to this day. And even in the industrialized West, American colonists and European farmers were starving to death as late as the 18th century. Having evolved under a near-constant threat of undernourishment and starvation, "your brain tells you that you should eat high-calorie foods whenever possible," says Andermann.

Fast-forward to the 21st century: factory farming, mass food processing and convenience culture give us access to hundreds of calories in a matter of seconds. But our "old brains haven't caught up to this new environment," says Andermann, and these once-helpful eating urges are backfiring. That said, we don't need to fear cravings, says dietitian Dana Notte, who specializes in treating women with life-

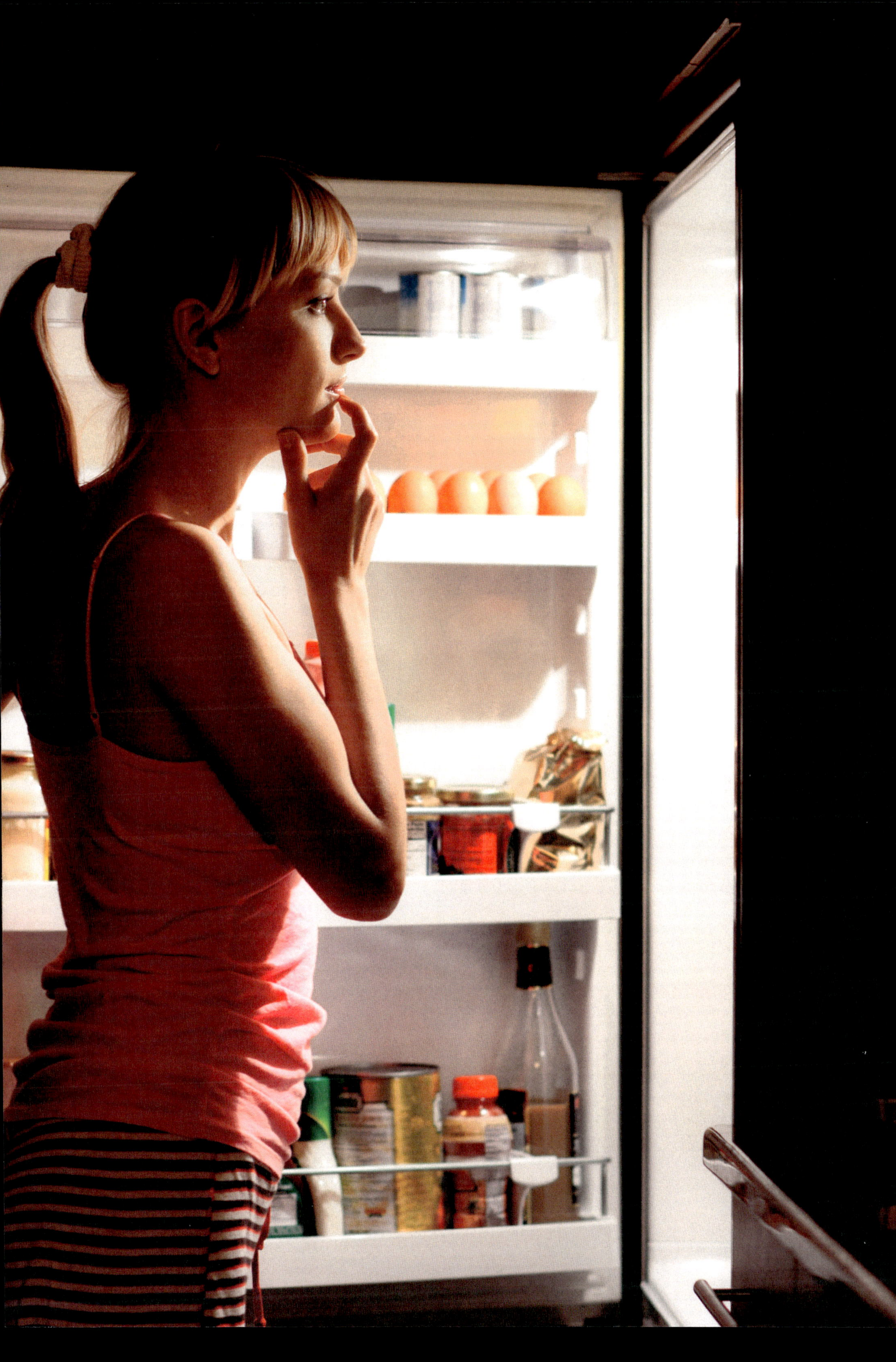

long weight struggles at Green Mountain at Fox Run, a mindful-eating retreat in Ludlow, Vt. "The more we understand cravings and examine the roots of our drive to eat, the more we can actively choose what to do with those cravings and take better care of our bodies."

Your craving brain

Food cravings originate in the brain, not just your belly. Hormones, memories, sights, smells, emotions, thoughts and signals between brain cells all influence what and how much you want to eat. For example, research shows that enticing images of food on billboards and TV trigger cravings and drive (over-) consumption, and these effects are even more pronounced when you're hungry. Directly after a meal, these "food cues" lose much of their punch, at least in average-weight individuals, says Andermann. But people with obesity or binge-eating issues don't experience that same steep post-meal drop-off, suggesting that brain differences may be at least partly responsible for some people's persistent cravings.

Cravings can change over time—especially if a person begins to eat a larger variety of nutritious foods.

Internal physical cues kick off cravings, too, but not in the way you may think. "Generally speaking, we don't have much evidence to support the idea that needs for specific vitamins or minerals trigger cravings for particular foods," says Notte. "What we do see in nutrient deficiency is the body encouraging you to go out and seek more food in general to try to fill in the gaps." Although you're not more likely to crave steak for the iron, cravings for sugars and carbohydrates soar when blood sugar drops, such as when you skip meals. "Carbohydrates are the body's preferred source of energy and the easiest to break down into glucose, so your body will seek them out when you need an energy boost," she says. Intake of carbohydrates spikes when we're sleep deprived.

Foods high in fat, sugar and certain other additives also cause sudden spikes in dopamine in parts of the brain related to "reward" and pleasure, explains Miguel Alonso-Alonso, director of the Laboratory of Bariatric and Nutritional Neuroscience at Beth Israel Deaconess Medical Center in Boston. Simply put, these "hyperpalatable" foods make us feel *gooood* in some of the very same ways that sex and drugs do. Whether sugar or any other food is literally, diagnosably "addictive" is still a matter of debate. What's not: reward signals in the brain can override cues like fullness in many people, contributing to overeating, weight gain and, sometimes, addict-like behavior around food, he says.

That said, cravings and food preferences can change over time—especially if a person begins to eat a larger variety of nutritious foods. Try to focus on what you're adding instead of what you're considering off-limits, says Notte. "Rather than approaching it as 'I really need to cut out white flour,' ask yourself what types of starches, such as whole grains and beans, you could add into your diet to bring more balance there. When we can bring more balance into our diet and meet our bodies' overall needs, we do start to see that our cravings change."

Giving in to every fatty, sugary food whim can cause weight gain, insulin resistance and other negative health outcomes. But actively ignoring and suppressing cravings can backfire, leading to a restrict-and-binge cycle (otherwise known as yo-yo dieting) that contributes to some of the very same health problems. "Cutting a food out of our diets generally increases cravings for that food—thinking a food is off-limits makes us want it so much more," says Notte. "It's the scarcity effect. Cravings and overeating behaviors are, in part, related to perceived food scarcity and uncertainty about when it'll be available again." Indeed, researchers have found that when mice are deprived of food for several hours and then are given access to a sugary liquid, they binge on it—whereas animals with constant access to the sugar don't. A similar rebound effect is seen in humans.

For most people with lifelong weight struggles, here's how that cycle plays out: Restricting calories and food groups increases cravings for off-limits foods. After a month or three months or a year, when a person's resolve breaks—as it nearly always does—he's probably going to overeat those high-calorie foods, even binge. For some folks, this "rebound eating" can go on for days, weeks or even months.

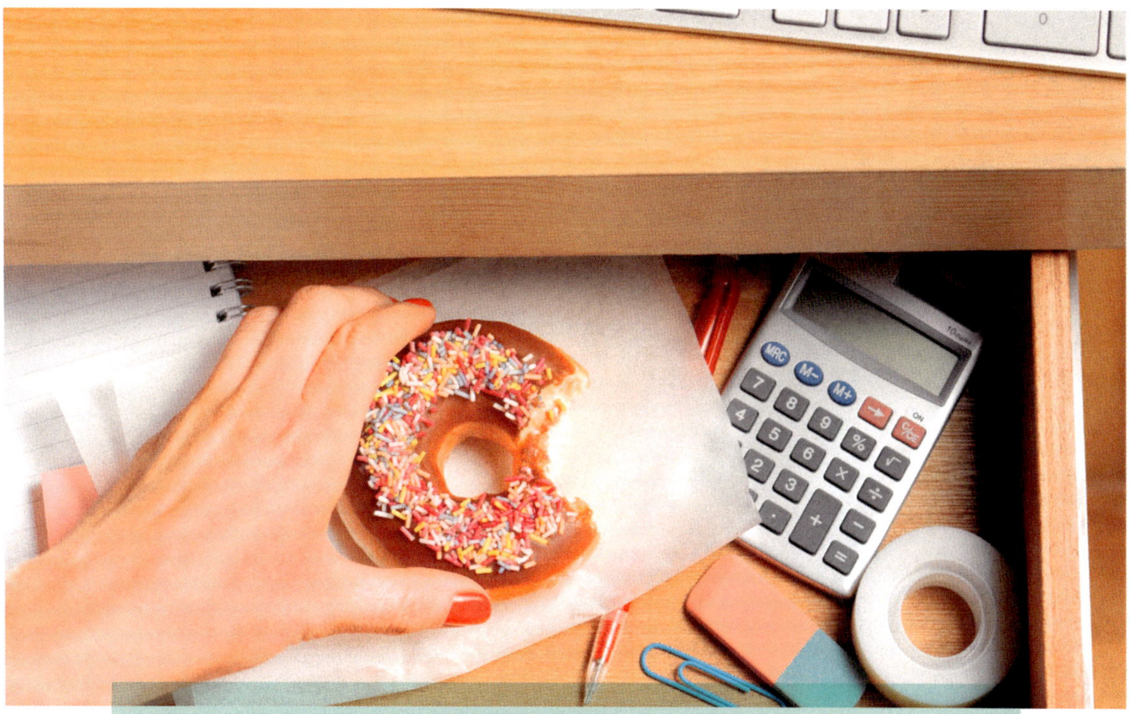

Tempted by treats at the office? Ask yourself: Am I truly hungry for this now? You may find you just need a mental break, like a walk or a chat with a co-worker.

Mindful habits

For most of human history, cravings and constant food seeking helped us survive lean times. But the modern foodscape is one of ubiquitous, cheap calories marketed to us by a $5 trillion food-retail industry. This is where the reasonable, prefrontal-cortex part of our big brains come in, says Andermann. We can tap this region to do three things: stop and notice cravings, decipher where they're coming from and choose how to respond. "When asked how they know when they're finished with a meal, Americans say it's when a TV show is over, or when their plates are empty—not when they feel full," says Andermann. "The first step in changing any kind of learned action is mindfulness—paying attention."

You might start by noticing what you're doing when a hankering crops up. Habits are a powerful trigger for cravings, says Alonso-Alonso. Our brains like convenience and efficiency above all else, and "habits operate as behavioral shortcuts in daily life and are a preferred mode of making decisions with minimal effort," he says. Shake up your routine as much as you can to create more of a pause between craving and action.

"Sometimes all you need is a moment to ask yourself if you're truly hungry for this right now," says Notte. You may realize that you're tired and what you need is to turn off the TV and go to bed. Or perhaps you're stressed, and the craving is more about soothing yourself than how yummy the food is. Folks with emotional- and binge-eating issues especially may crave certain foods as a kind of self-medication, says Andermann. Cognitive behavioral therapy (CBT) and dialectical behavioral therapy (DBT) are both research-backed ways people with emotional cravings can gain more control over their eating behaviors.

Regular physical activity has also been linked to a greater ability to actively control eating behavior. Animal studies suggest it could be due to changes in blood flow, the release of certain brain chemicals such as feel-good endorphins and better functioning of neurons, says Alonso-Alonso.

The answer to "Why am I craving this food?" may simply be that you want the pleasure of eating it. That's OK, insists Notte. "Your ultimate goal should never be simply to not eat the food that you're craving," she says. Instead, the aim is to make a mindful and informed decision that balances your needs in the moment with what you want in the long term. "Food is a great pleasure," she continues, "and humans are pleasure-seeking creatures. Sometimes just allowing ourselves to enjoy the food and then move on really is the best way to handle it." □

14 Healthy Foods That Keep You Full

Reach for one of these hunger-busting picks, and you won't find yourself reaching for a cookie an hour later

> ***By Kathleen Felton***

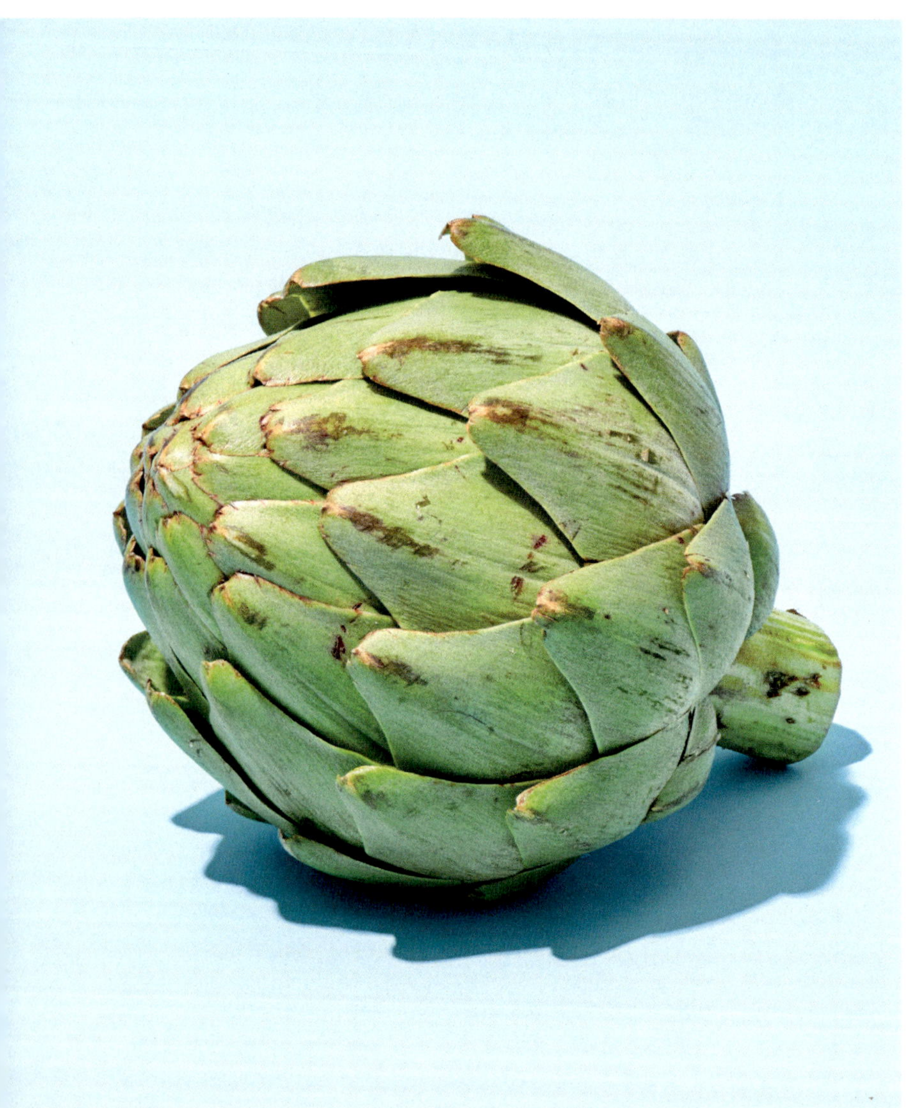

Artichokes

Artichokes are super filling—in fact, they are one of the highest-fiber vegetables. A single boiled artichoke has 10.3 grams of fiber—almost half the recommended daily amount for women.

Dark chocolate

Dark chocolate contains monounsaturated fatty acids that could help speed up your metabolism, says Cynthia Sass, RD. "I love to chop dark chocolate into squares and add them into a smoothie."

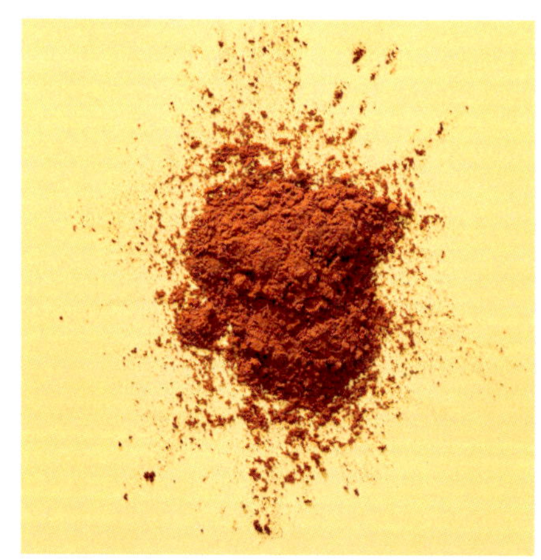

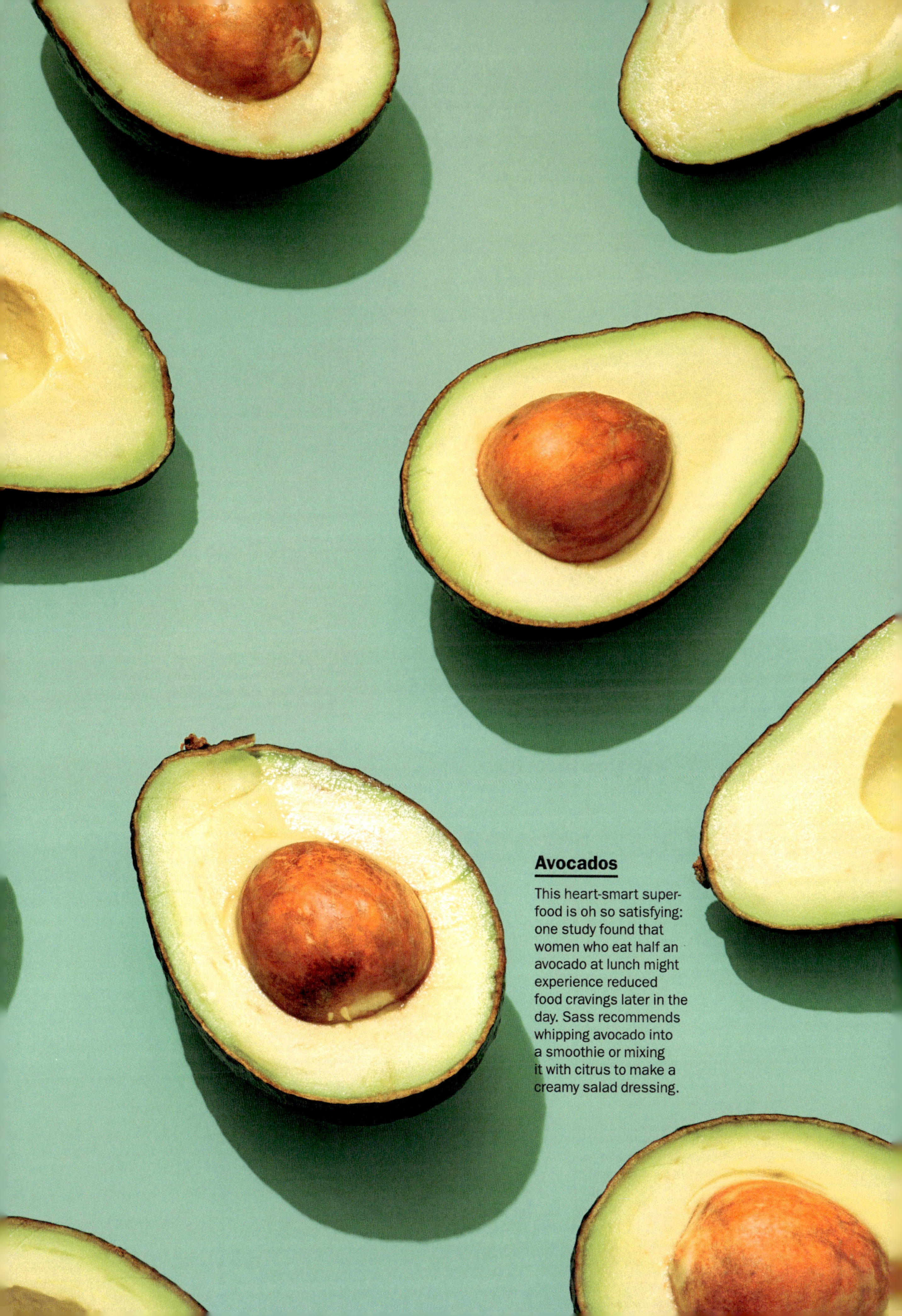

Avocados

This heart-smart superfood is oh so satisfying: one study found that women who eat half an avocado at lunch might experience reduced food cravings later in the day. Sass recommends whipping avocado into a smoothie or mixing it with citrus to make a creamy salad dressing.

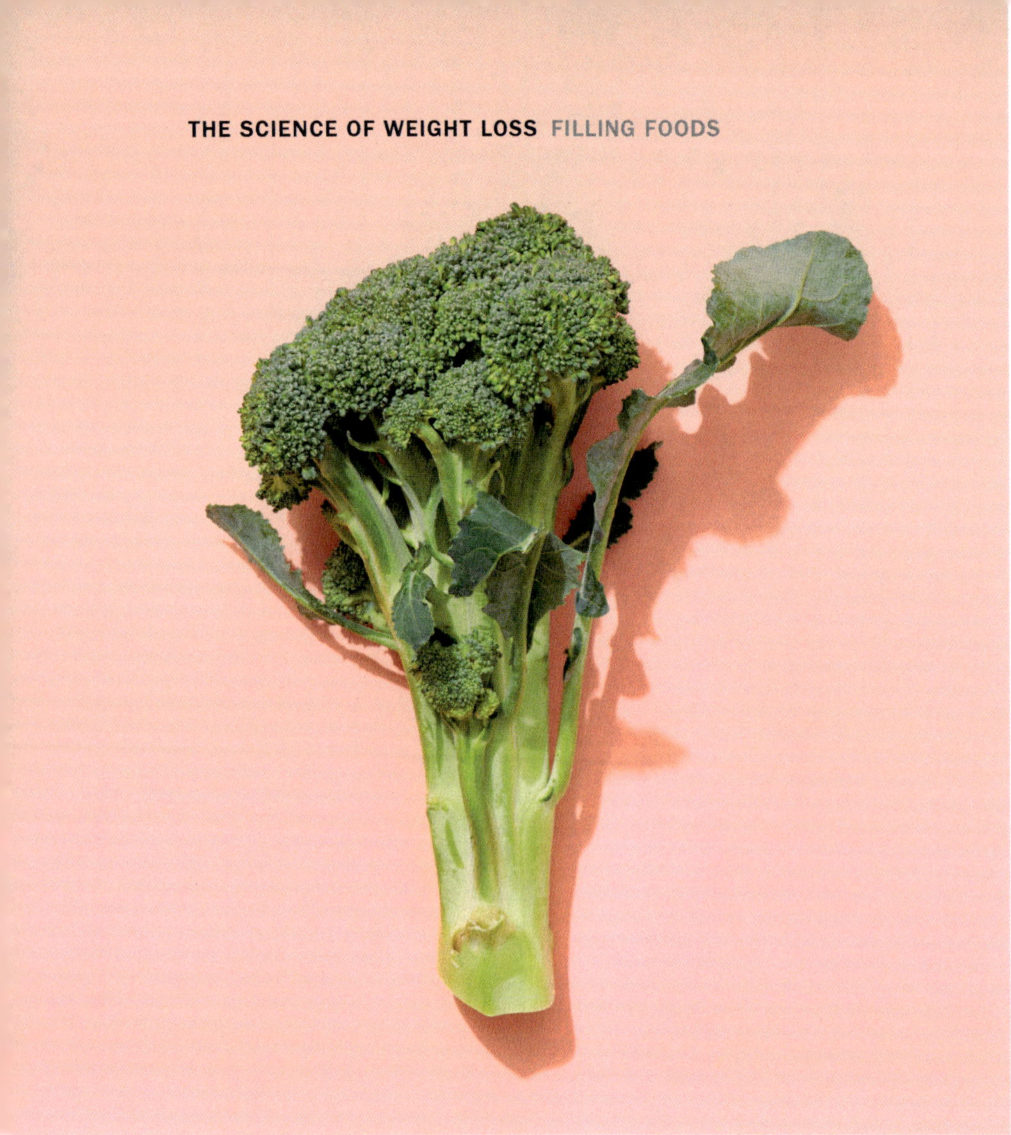

Broccoli

A mighty source of calcium and important cancer-fighting compounds, broccoli also has loads of filling fiber and will set you back only 30 calories per serving. If this cruciferous veggie makes you bloat, steam it first to make it easier to digest.

Eggs

You might not think of them as a weight-loss food, but eggs are packed with protein, which helps curb your appetite. One study found that overweight women who ate eggs for breakfast lost twice as much weight as women who started their days with bagels.

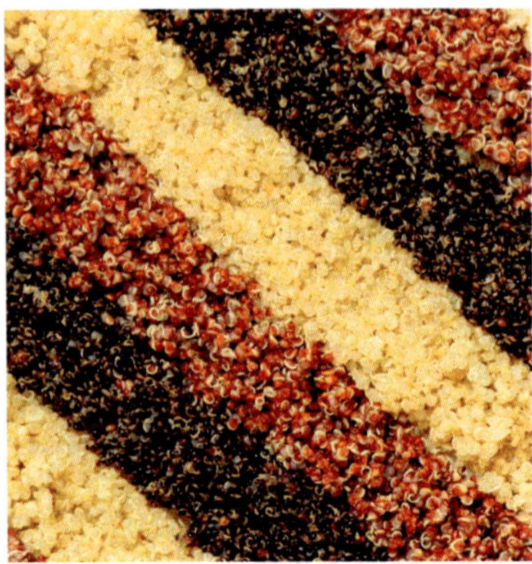

Quinoa

Quinoa contains hearty doses of iron and magnesium, which help give your body energy. And a one-cup serving of this seed boasts 8 grams of filling protein and 5 grams of fiber. Confused about how to cook quinoa? It's delicious in a salad, in burger patties or pancakes, or baked into muffins.

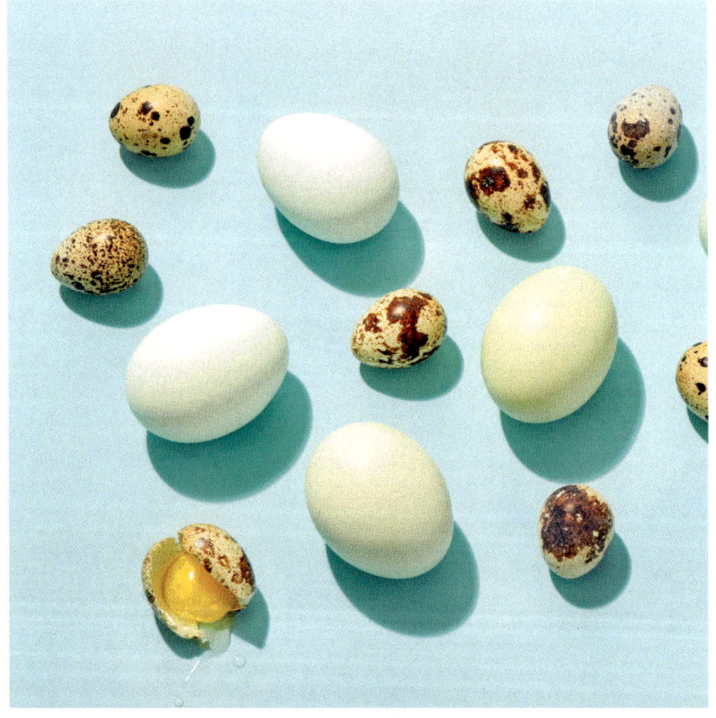

Almonds

Almonds are light (just 163 calories for 23). In one study, people who added a daily serving of them to a low-cal diet lost more weight than those who ate a carb-rich snack such as crackers.

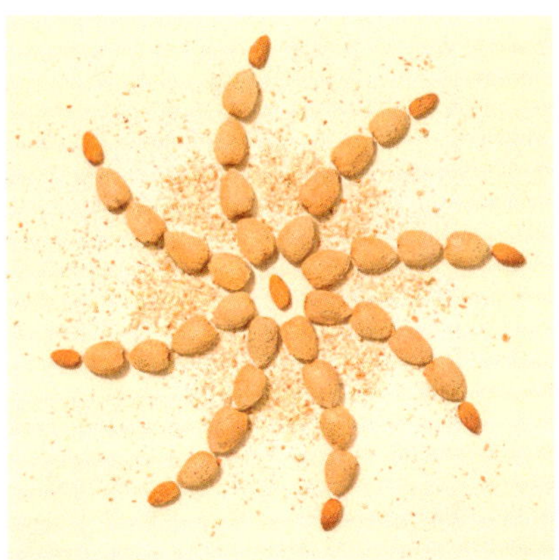

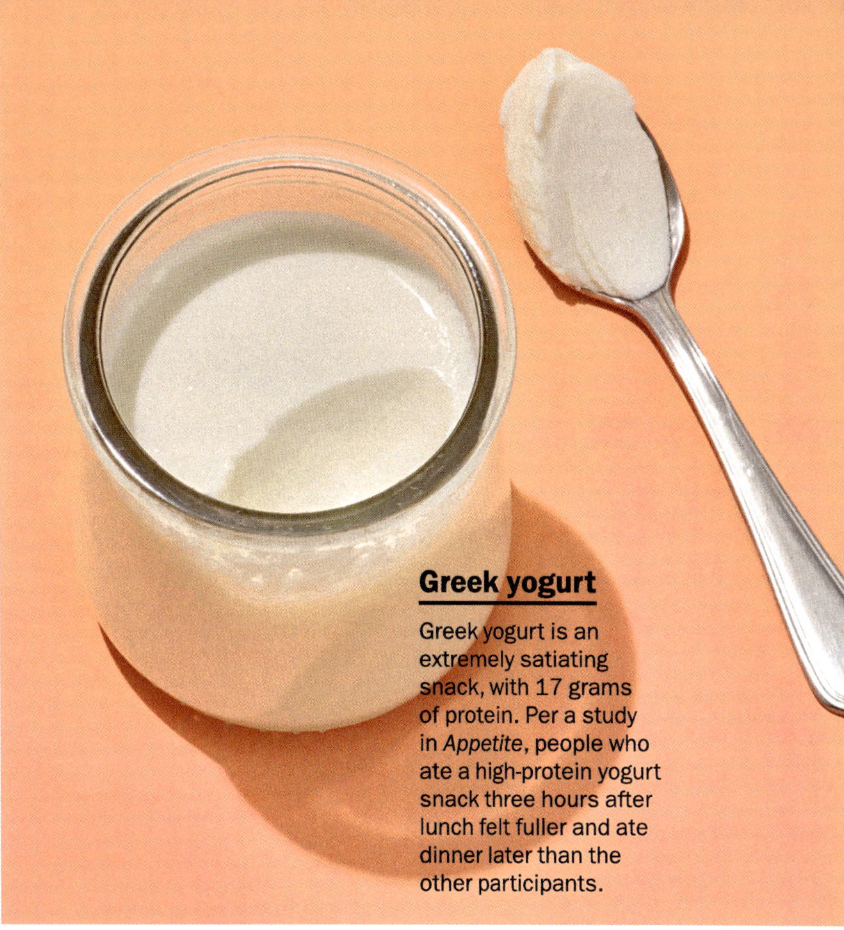

Greek yogurt

Greek yogurt is an extremely satiating snack, with 17 grams of protein. Per a study in *Appetite*, people who ate a high-protein yogurt snack three hours after lunch felt fuller and ate dinner later than the other participants.

Popcorn

With the exception of movie popcorn—which can pack 1,000 calories or more—popcorn is a healthy, filling snack. "In addition to all of the benefits of being a member of the whole-grain family, popcorn is light and airy, so you can eat a large portion," says Sass.

Lentils

There's a reason lentils are considered one of the world's healthiest foods. With 13 grams of protein and 11 grams of fiber per serving, this legume will keep you feeling full for hours in between meals. They're a great source of fat-burning resistant starch, too, with 3.4 grams in a half-cup serving. Lentils also boast twice as much iron as other legumes and are especially good sources of vitamin B and folate.

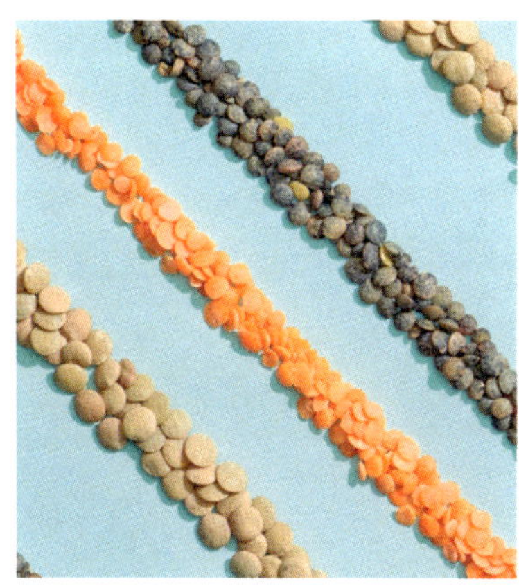

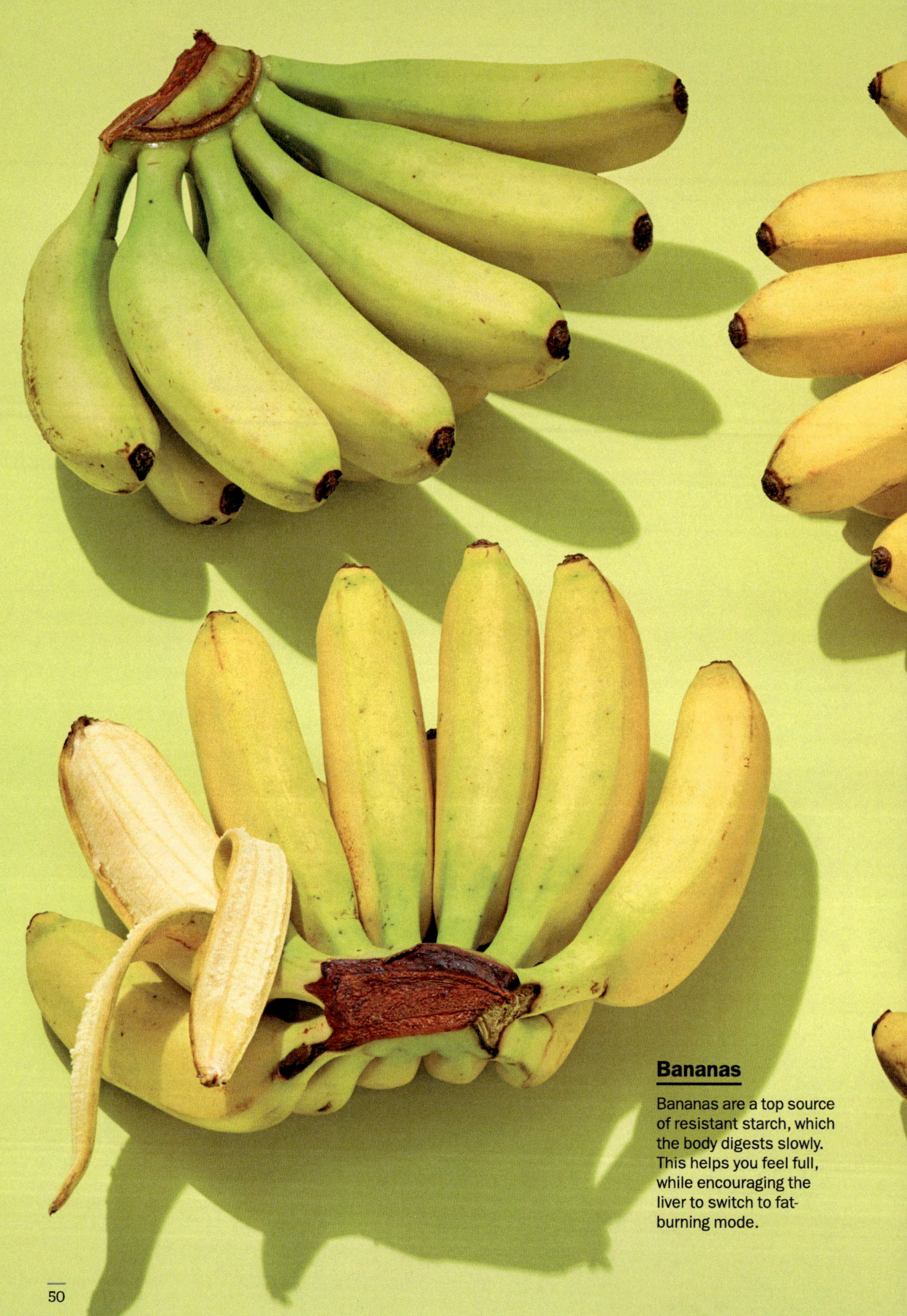

Bananas

Bananas are a top source of resistant starch, which the body digests slowly. This helps you feel full, while encouraging the liver to switch to fat-burning mode.

Chia seeds

Small-but-mighty chia seeds pack a serious fiber punch—4 grams per tablespoon—so when you add them to your favorite healthy foods, they'll help ward off hunger.

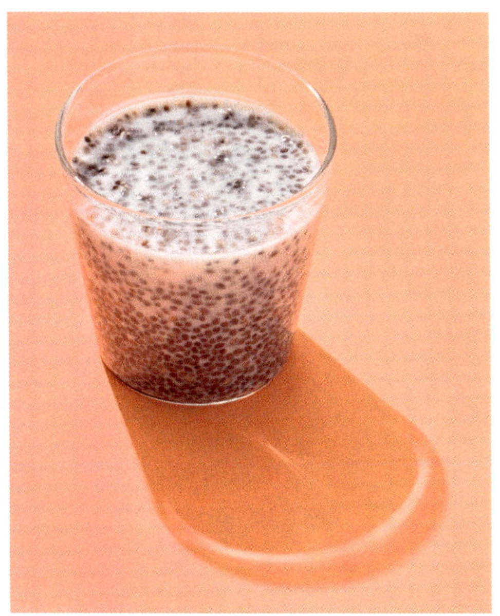

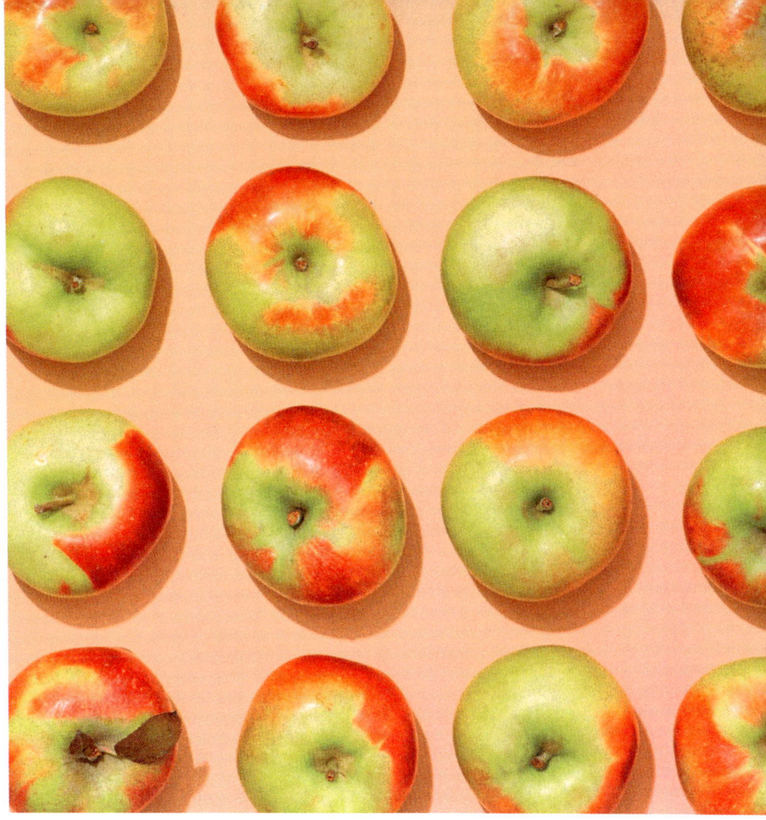

Apples

Apples have pectin, which slows digestion and makes you feel full. Research shows eating a whole apple with your meal (versus drinking apple juice) is a natural appetite suppressant.

Oatmeal

Oats are another great source of resistant starch. In one study, people who ate hot oatmeal for breakfast felt less hunger later in the day than those who ate cold oat cereal.

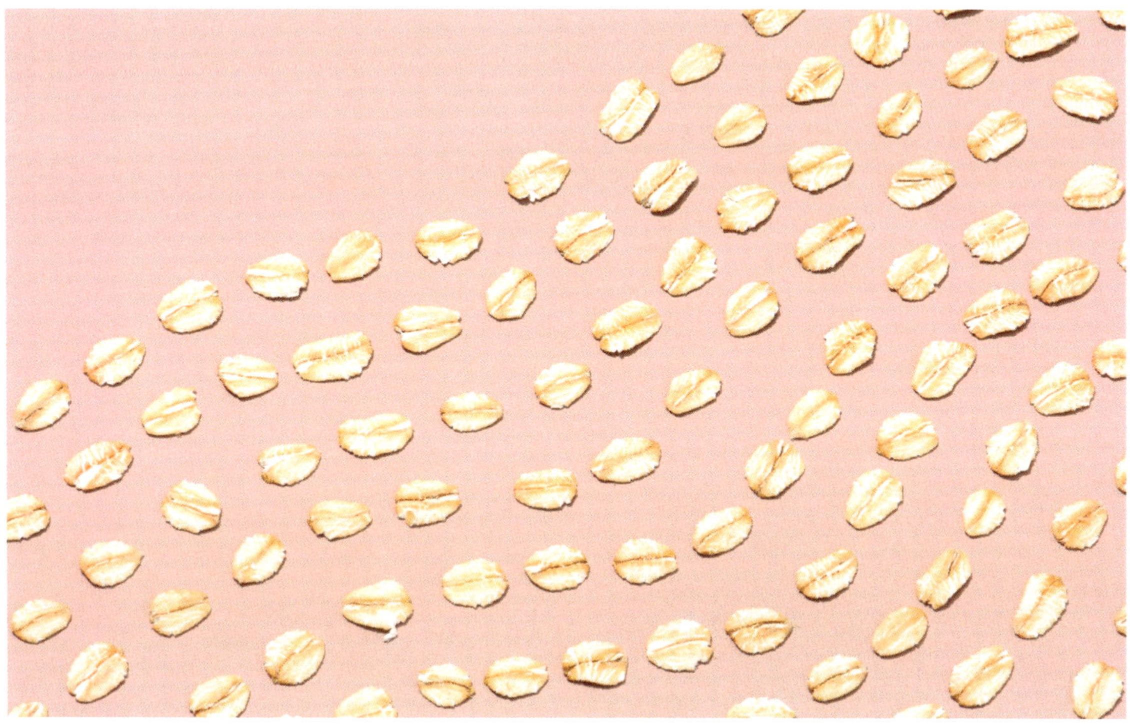

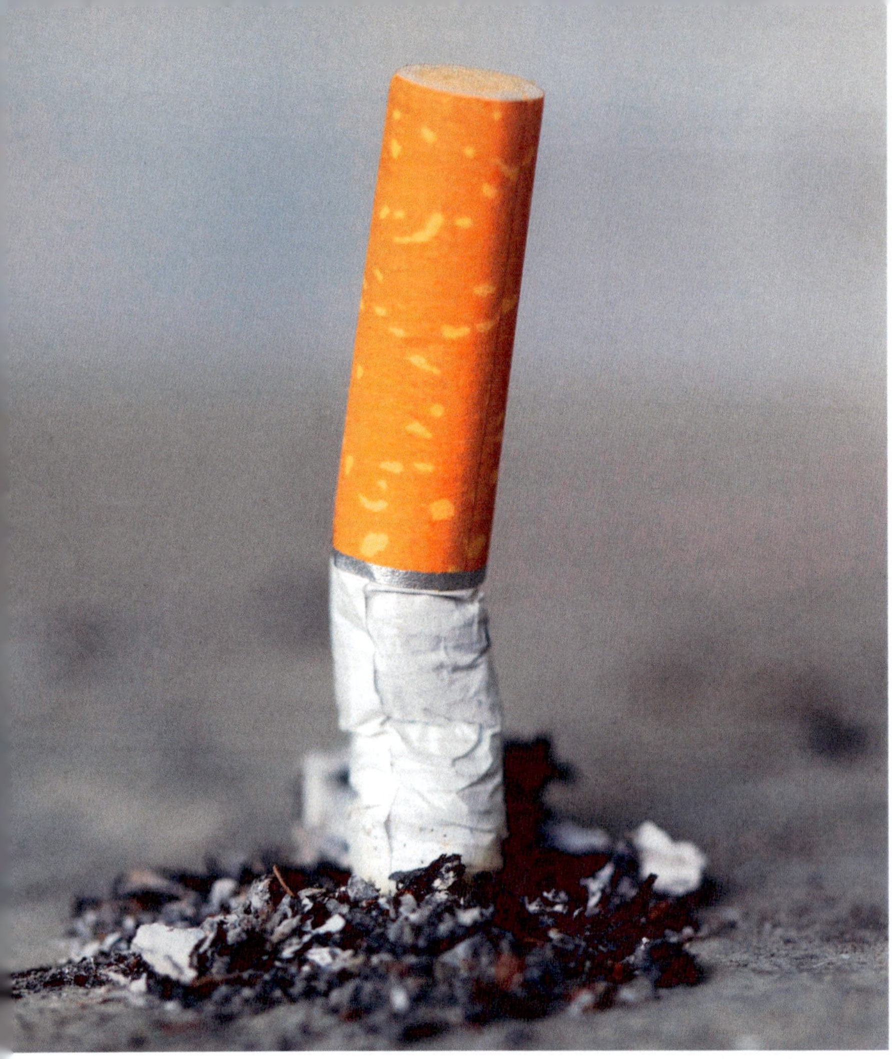

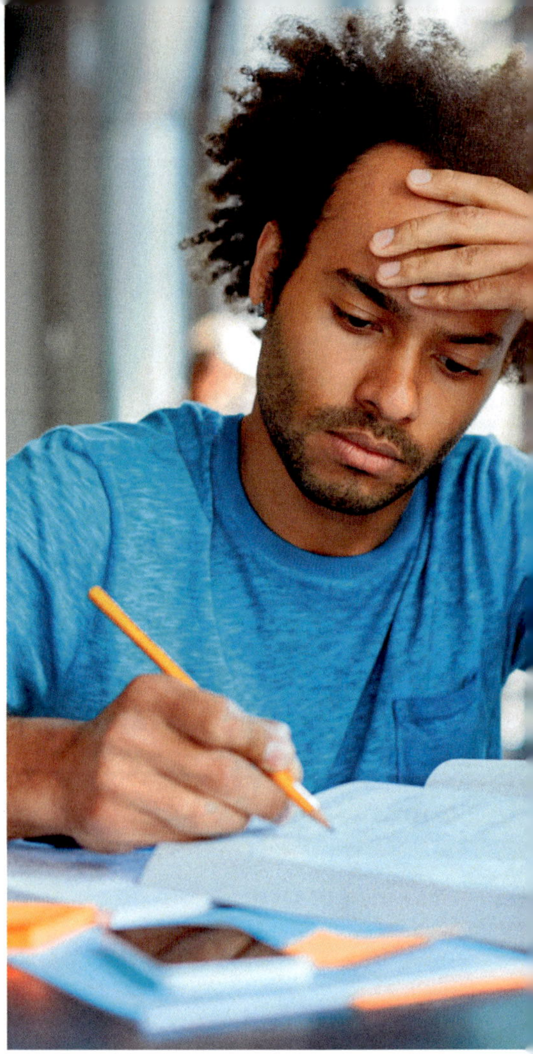

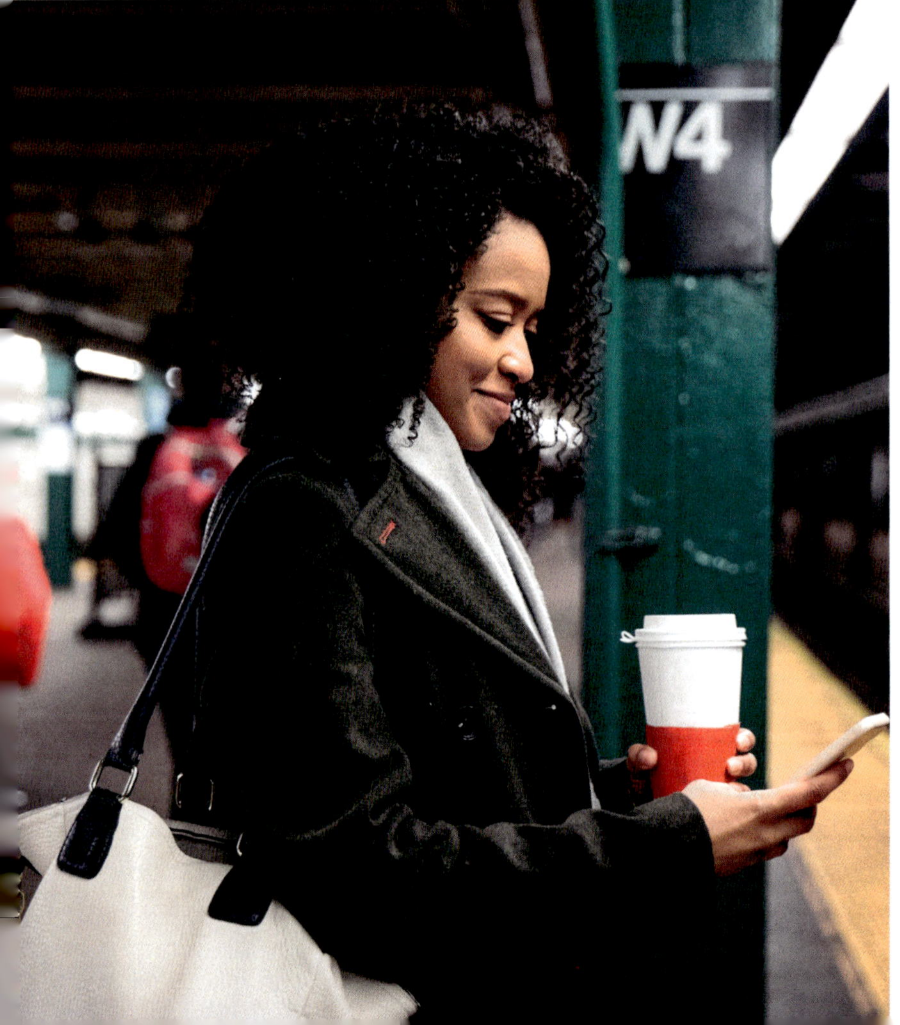

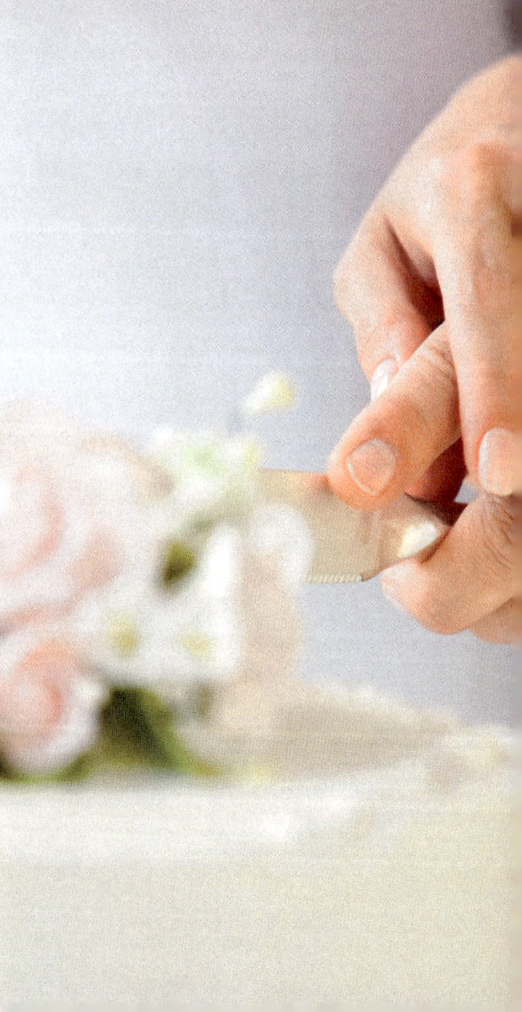

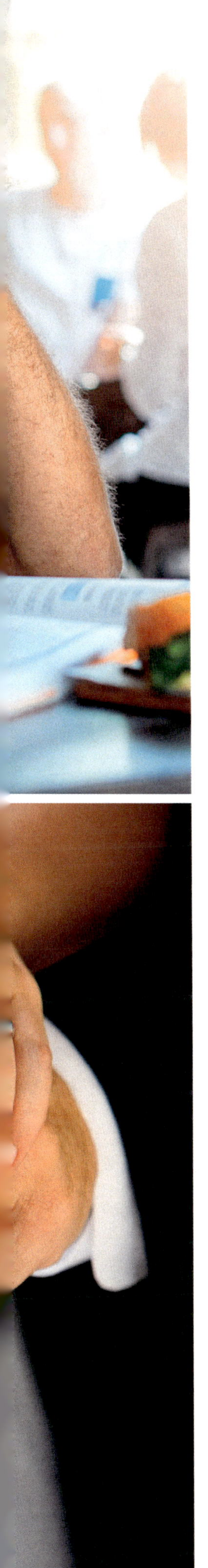

Gain-Proof Every Stage of Your Life

Ever notice how weight tends to creep on at certain times? Here's how to push through these vulnerable periods and come out healthier

> **By Jessica Migala**

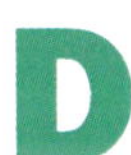

DESPITE WHAT YOU MAY HEAR, PEOPLE AREN'T DESIGNED to stay their exact same weight their entire adult lives. "Our bodies are changing all the time in relation to our environment," says Linda Bacon, a researcher and the author of *Body Respect*. "There are many things that factor into a changing weight over time, including a new environment or aging."

And while it may not feel great—we are conditioned to believe that thinner is better—you don't have to live in fear. Remember that you don't have to be a certain weight to eat a nutritious diet and get the recommended 150 minutes a week of moderate activity. "We can all adopt good health behaviors, regardless of what size we're at," says Bacon. Here's how to make it through five stages when weight problems often develop.

Tricky time: College

The theory goes that once you head off to college, midnight pizza-heavy study sessions, too many beers and free rein at the buffet at the dining hall pack on pounds (sometimes known as the "Freshman 15"). But—deep breath—it's probably not 15 pounds. A meta-analysis of 22 studies published in the journal *BMC Obesity* found that about 60% of students gained an average of 7.5 pounds during their freshman year.

It's a trend experts see in both men and women. "Weight tends to naturally trend up after high school, and I see this especially pronounced in men," says Benjamin O'Donnell, an endocrinologist specializing in weight management at the Ohio State University Wexner Medical Center. Men may be active in sports in high school, and when they get to college, they're not on a team anymore but "they don't stop eating like a football player," he says.

Of course, the same happens to women too; they're no longer on the field-hockey team but they're eating as if they're doing suicide sprints every day.

Young students may find that this is the first time in their life when they have food freedom, says Tracy Lockwood Beckerman, a registered dietitian in New York City. "Your normal eating habits become flipped, and you're dealing with the influence of new friends, a new schedule, stress and a new living situation."

The best way to avoid bulking up in college is to not focus on weight gain but instead focus on developing healthy new habits. It's unlikely that downing beer and pizza and staying up until 3 a.m. is living your best life, even if it feels fun at the time.

Everything may be new, but now's the time to develop stress-reduction strategies and get adequate sleep to buffer late-night binges. If you do find yourself face-to-face with midnight nachos, assemble a small plate of them so you don't mindlessly devour the order. Another suggestion for snack attacks: "Keep in-shell pistachios in your dorm room," she says. "The nuts require legwork to crack open, so you can't inhale them quickly."

Couples who are in happier, more supportive marriages stay at a healthier weight from the newlywed period into midlife.

Tricky time: Your early 20s

Going from college to career often means taking a desk job and enduring something of a commute. So it's probably no wonder that young adults add about a pound or two per year, per 2013 data from the Agency for Healthcare Research and Quality. In an effort to control this creeping weight gain—or strive for a certain body ideal—you may respond by trying to go on a diet. For all your good intentions, the strategy can backfire, leaving you with more fat than you had before. (We're not talking about attempts to eat healthy and balanced, but rather active efforts to restrict what you're eating.) In fact, adults who had a history of dieting were more likely to have gained weight over a 10-year period compared with those who ate regularly, according to a 2018 study in the journal *Eating Behaviors*.

When you shortchange your body of calories (energy), it stimulates physiological mechanisms that amplify hunger and add body fat; psychologically speaking, drastic diets also make you hyper-focus on food, increasing the likelihood of a binge, says Bacon. This is often what leads to regaining more weight than you had lost.

What you can do: "It's important for people to know that dieting doesn't get them what it promises," says Bacon. "If you want to get to a weight that's healthy for you, the idea isn't to try to control or fight your body but trust it."

Tuning in to your body through things like intuitive eating (in which you honor your hunger and cravings without relying on restriction) puts your body back in the driver's seat.

Next, ask yourself how you can fit exercise into your workday. Could you do 15 minutes of a streaming workout at home? Is there an office park you can walk around at lunch? Getting regular exercise not only makes it easier to keep weight steady but also lowers your risk of many serious health problems.

Tricky time: Early married life

Did you come back from your honeymoon feeling a little puffy? It's not just you: the transition into married life leads to weight gain in men and women, according to a 2012 study review from researchers at the City University of New York. (Interestingly, the transition out of marriage leads to weight loss, the CUNY researchers found.) One Finnish study they looked at, for example, found that both men and women who transitioned into marriage almost doubled their risk of substantial weight gain compared with consistently married people. The CUNY experts theorized that couples may be eating more together, moving less and not worrying so much about their looks once they become locked in.

In some cases, they're just putting back the weight that they crash dieted off before walking down the aisle. ("Sweating for the wedding" is a thing, after all.) Problem is, the extreme methods people try to get slim fast to fit into their wedding dress or tux are unsustainable. "If you dieted to the extreme, that weight will come back on after the wedding, since it's an unrealistic vision for where your body should have been," says Beckerman. "Your body is fighting to go back to a weight more in line with its genetic set point."

First off, don't crash diet before the wedding. It will leave you vulnerable to binge eating and developing a negative relationship with food. Once you're hitched, if you're a healthy eater and your mate isn't, "don't feel trapped in your partner's eating habits just because you're a duo," Beckerman says. Take turns cooking and you may just convert your spouse to loving grain bowls and grilled fish. Focusing on your relationship can pay off too. Research shows that couples in happier, more supportive marriages stay at a healthier weight from the newlywed period into midlife.

Tricky time: New motherhood

It's not OK to expect a woman postpartum to "snap back" to her former body. The things you did to maintain the weight you were at B.K. (that's before kids) likely aren't your priorities anymore now that there's a little one to care for. "After having a baby, your routine has been flipped on its head," says Beckerman.

Although there's no reason to feel pressure to regain your old shape, some women put healthy eating habits on the back burner for years after starting their family, which can lead to problems down the road. One study on women who entered pregnancy with a normal BMI discovered that one third became overweight or obese a year postpartum, per the journal *Obstetrics & Gynecology*. This of course has health implications, as excess weight can put a woman at risk for heart disease, diabetes and some cancers.

So what's a healthy way to address those new-mom pounds? Six months postpartum, think about how you can start to shift your habits—and it doesn't have to be an entire overhaul. Rather than focusing only on diet and exercise, put your efforts (and any limited free time) toward sleep. "Sleep deprivation can alter hormones responsible for hunger and fullness cues," says Beckerman.

In addition, give yourself grace during this very stressful period. "Don't be so hard on yourself," she adds. "If you can relieve the pressure to be perfect and that thinner is better, you can really shift your thinking toward how certain foods will make you feel instead of how they will make you look." To make healthier eating easier on yourself, consider signing up for a meal-kit delivery service that sends pre-prepped ingredients with recipes to make it simpler to throw together a balanced dinner.

Try thinking of every meal as an opportunity to make a healthy choice. Go with lean protein, whole grains and at least five servings a day of fruits and vegetables. But don't beat yourself up if you have an off meal. So you ate three cookies for lunch while standing over the sink! No one is perfect. Dinner will provide another chance to eat right.

Tricky time: Quitting smoking

You may be hesitant to give up cigarettes because you're worried you will put on pounds after quitting. "When you quit smoking, you can expect some amount of weight gain because nicotine suppresses appetite," says O'Donnell. Some people gain 10 to 20 pounds, he adds. Ex-smokers may feel hungrier and also find that they're scarfing down snacks because they're so accustomed to holding something in their hands.

O'Donnell recommends that recent quitters find a no-calorie substitute, such as sugar-free chewing gum or naturally flavored carbonated water, that keeps their mouth busy and fills the void left by cigarettes. It's also a good idea to have healthy snacks on hand, so you're reaching for carrots and hummus or an apple instead of a big bag of chips.

And even if the scale does tick up, rest assured that you will be healthier in the long run—even if you're heavier. While the risk of Type 2 diabetes rose in the short term among recent quitters who gained weight, their hearts were still healthier for it. Even people who gained more than 20 pounds lowered their odds of dying from cardiovascular disease by 67% compared with ongoing smokers, according to a 2018 study in *The New England Journal of Medicine*.

As O'Donnell says, "Remind yourself that you're doing something positive for your health." □

Eat Out and Stay Lean

Yes, you can enjoy restaurant meals without putting on pounds. Here's how to find the best bets on any menu

> By Courtney Mifsud

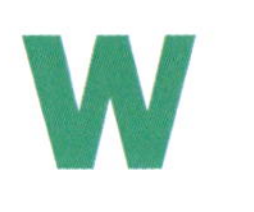

WHEN IT COMES TO EATING HEALTHY, IT'S MUCH EASier when you're in your own kitchen. Baked chicken instead of fried? Check. Whole grains instead of refined pasta? Deal. But so many of our best eating intentions get sabotaged when we step into a typical restaurant. Behind the scenes, simple appetizers plunge into deep fryers, pan-seared fillets of fish are basted with butter, and sugar sneaks in where you least expect it.

In 2017, the American Heart Association unveiled a yearlong study that confirmed what most of us have suspected for years: diets go off the rails when people eat out. The study followed 150 overweight people who were already on weight-loss plans. Study participants checked in on a smartphone app multiple times a day and reported whether they had strayed from the plan, noting where they were as well as who they were with. Not surprisingly, participants reported the most temptations when they were at a bar or restaurant and around other people eating. "You might think that everybody knows they're at higher risk when they go into a restaurant, but people go out into these toxic environments and they forget," the study's lead author, Lora Burke, a professor of nursing at the University of Pittsburgh, told TIME in 2017. "We remind people that it's not a diet they can go on and off; it's a lifestyle," she said.

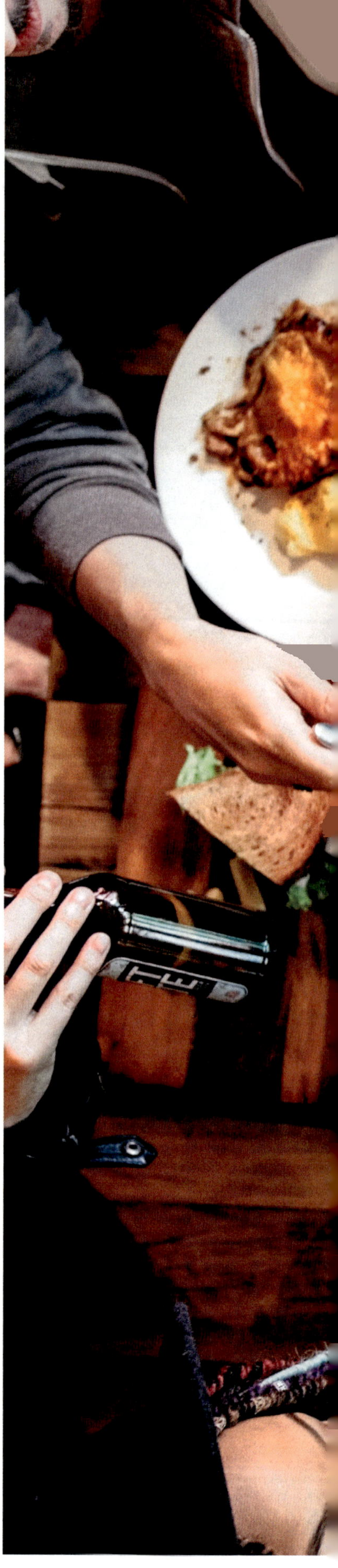

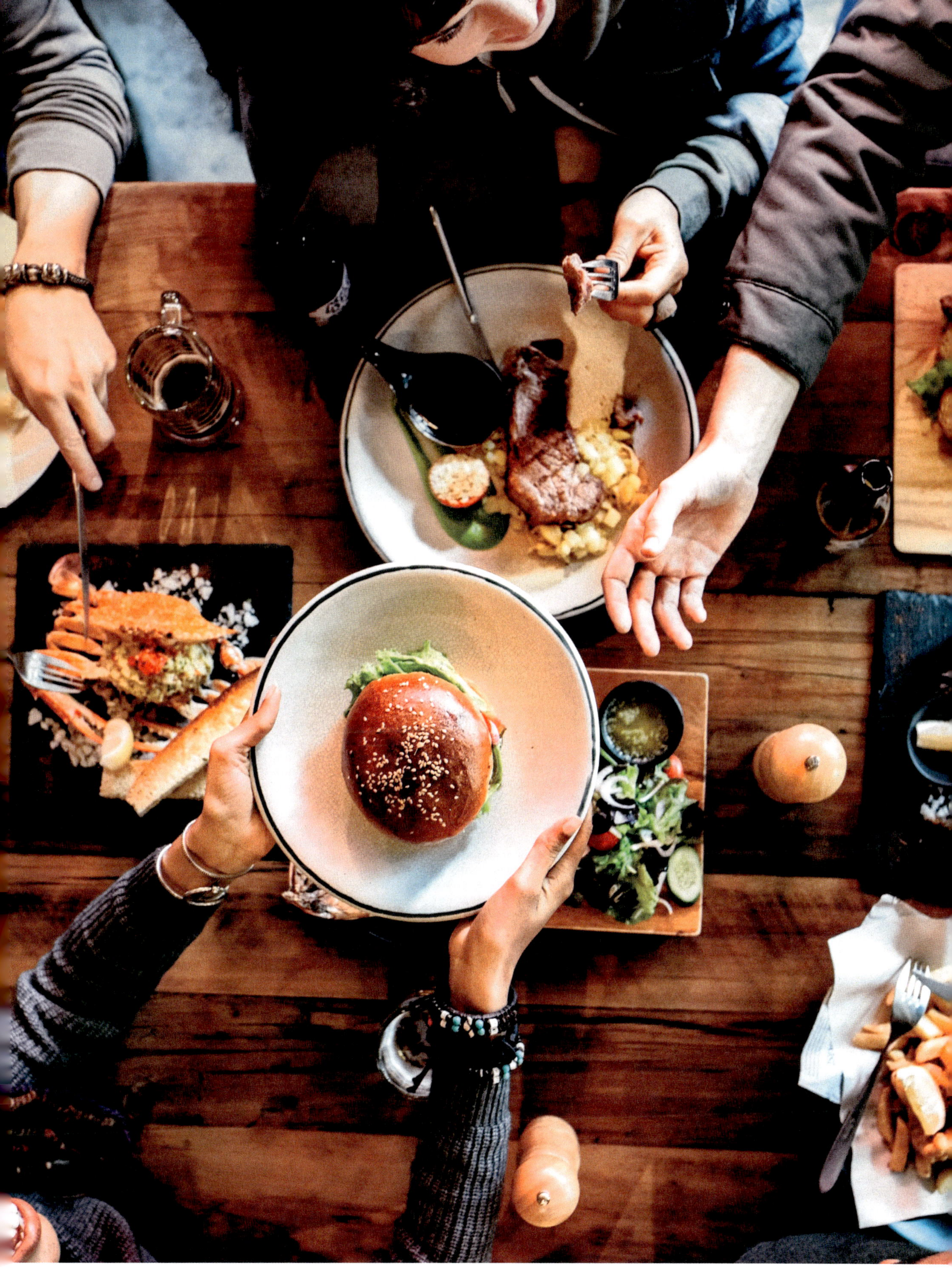

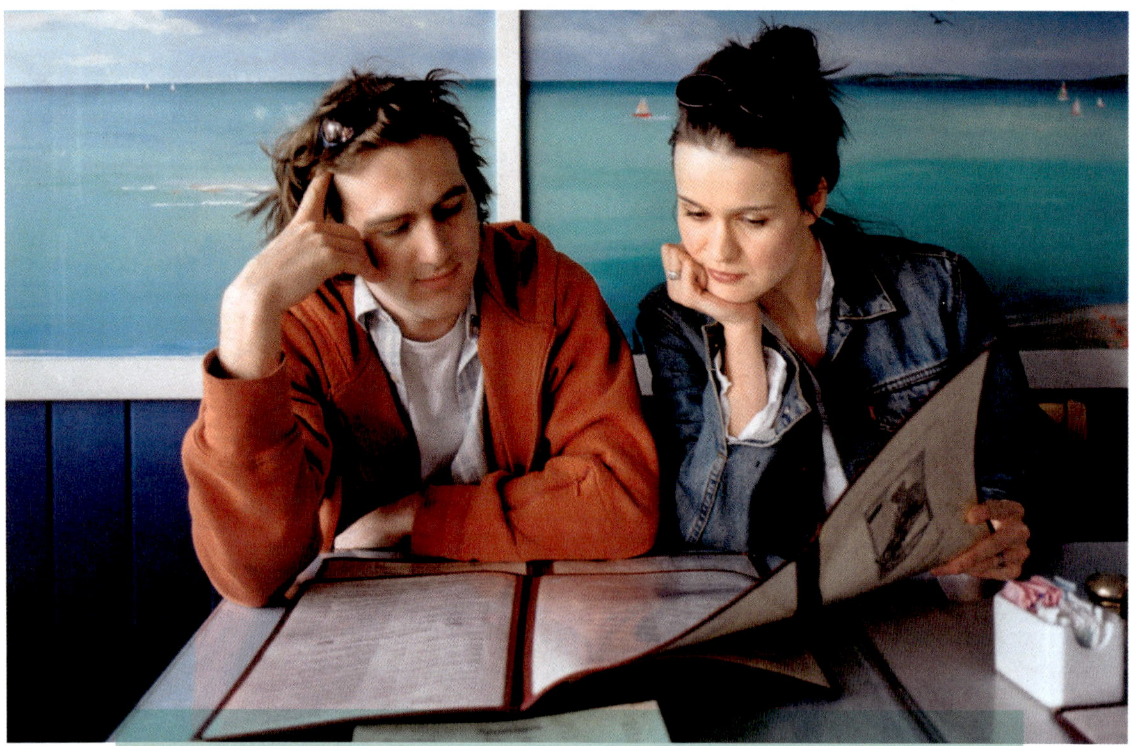

Scanning the menu? Be on the lookout for code words like "creamy," "rich" and "juicy"—they signal fattening fare and encourage diners to overindulge.

"It's OK if they want to go out Friday night and eat wings, but then they need to cut back on Thursday and Saturday."

The temptations of a restaurant begin when you walk in the door. Researchers at the University of California, Berkeley, found evidence that merely smelling food could lead to weight gain. In their 2017 study, mice were split into three groups: one group had their usual sense of smell, one had their sense of smell shut off, and a third set was given a heightened sense of smell. These mice all ate the same high-fat diet, and while they all gained weight, the greater the sense of smell, the more weight they gained. Once the heavier mice in the third group had their scent superpowers shut off, they dropped the weight.

That's not to suggest that any of us should wear nose plugs when sitting down to a meal out. Instead, just be aware of how heavenly smells can affect appetite. A 30-minute wait standing near the kitchen, with the aroma of a freshly cooked steak and garlicky french fries wafting through the air, could trigger you to eat more than you would have if you sat right down at your table. Making a reservation in advance can help minimize the aroma effect.

Once you get to your table, there's a way to make choices that align with your goals. If you know the restaurant ahead of time, preparation is your friend. Take a look at the menu online and decode some of the language. Descriptive emotion-rich adjectives like "creamy," "rich" and "juicy" are all over restaurant menus, and, according to Brian Wansink, the author of *Mindless Eating*, these words can seduce diners. Wansink found that descriptive labels increased sales by as much as 27% and nudged people toward a restaurant purchase they might not have otherwise made. By mulling over the menu from your laptop instead of in the moment, you'll have time to consider your options without impulse and go with more nourishing picks.

A 2015 study in the *Journal of the American Academy of Nutrition and Dietetics* also backs up how unhealthy restaurant meals can be. According to the study, a staggering 92% of meals from large-chain and local restaurants had more than the recommended calories for the average person for a single meal. The researchers found that portion sizes in the restaurant industry are obscene. "Some meals exceeded the calories recommended for a whole day," Susan Roberts, director of the Energy Metabolism Laboratory at the Jean Mayer USDA Human Nutrition Research Center on Aging at Tufts University, told TIME in 2016. "Our biology is designed to make us eat when there's food there. I don't think anybody should feel bad that they get weak when there's an excessive portion in front of them, because the problem is the excessive portion, not them."

There are strategies to help you avoid polishing off a steak as big as your head or an omelet fit for three. Consider splitting an entrée with your partner or friend; you can even add a healthy appetizer or a veggie-rich salad to your shared meal to bulk up its nutritional content.

Supersized indeed: 92% of restaurant meals exceed the recommended calories for the average person, one study found.

Another way around the portion distortion is to ask the server to box up half of your meal to go and bring you only the remaining half. Ordering two appetizers instead of an entrée is a favorite trick of dietitians. If you go with tuna tartare and a side salad, for instance, you get a balanced mix of protein, healthy fats and healthy carbs without a lot of calories. As a general rule, avoid fried appetizers like jalapeño poppers and anything covered in cheese. According to Mike Moreno, the author of *The 17 Day Diet*, some fried apps pack the amount of fat that four people should have in a whole day.

Salads may seem like the ultimate healthy order, but they can add unwanted calories and absurd amounts of saturated fat. In chain restaurants in particular, meal salads tend to come in an oversize bowl, packed with fattening extras like bacon, croutons and fried strips of chicken. Taco salads are especially likely to derail healthy-eating intentions. Often served in a fried tortilla shell with a bed of iceberg lettuce rather than mixed greens, they are loaded with saturated fat (from sour cream, cheese, ground beef, etc.) without giving you much in the way of vegetables. Look for a salad that contains a lean protein such as chicken, salmon, edamame or chickpeas, ideally one source of fat (think avocado or cheese) and nutritious extras such as mushrooms or plain (that is, not candied) nuts.

Salad dressing can be a source of healthy fats—or a creamy, calorie-laden disaster. Going with olive oil and balsamic vinegar or a squeeze of lemon rather than prepared dressings gives you flavor without too many excess calories. You're best off staying away from low-fat dressings, though. Although they may seem like a diet-friendly sub, these options aren't as healthy as you might think. A 2012 Purdue University study examined salads dressed with various types of fat and found that different levels of fat in the dressing limited the benefits of the salad. "In order to get more from eating fruits and vegetables, they need to be paired correctly with fat-based dressings," said Mario Ferruzzi, the study's lead author. "While a salad with fat-free dressing is lower in calories, the absence of fat causes the loss of some of the benefits of eating vegetables."

And did you know that your anxiety level when eating out also impacts your ability to stick to your goals? Navigating a stressful meal out like a first date or business lunch prompts many of us to order things that we normally wouldn't have. Instead of anxious ordering, if you find yourself stressed at the table, excuse yourself and take 5 to 10 deep breaths. Mindful breathing can move your body into a more relaxed state, which will allow you to make thoughtful food choices.

Finally, keep in mind that how you talk about food—to others and to yourself—can help you stick with healthy-eating goals. In a study published in the *Journal of Consumer Research*, dieters who said "I don't eat that" instead of "I can't eat that" when faced with temptations were more successful at resisting treats and more likely to choose a healthy snack. The researchers theorized that saying the words "I don't" lends a feeling of self-control rather than the forced deprivation implied by "I can't."

So when the dessert cart comes around or your friend is asking you to split an order of fried onion rings, try saying, "I don't eat that." You may find that those four simple words help you stick with your goal—and feel happy about it. □

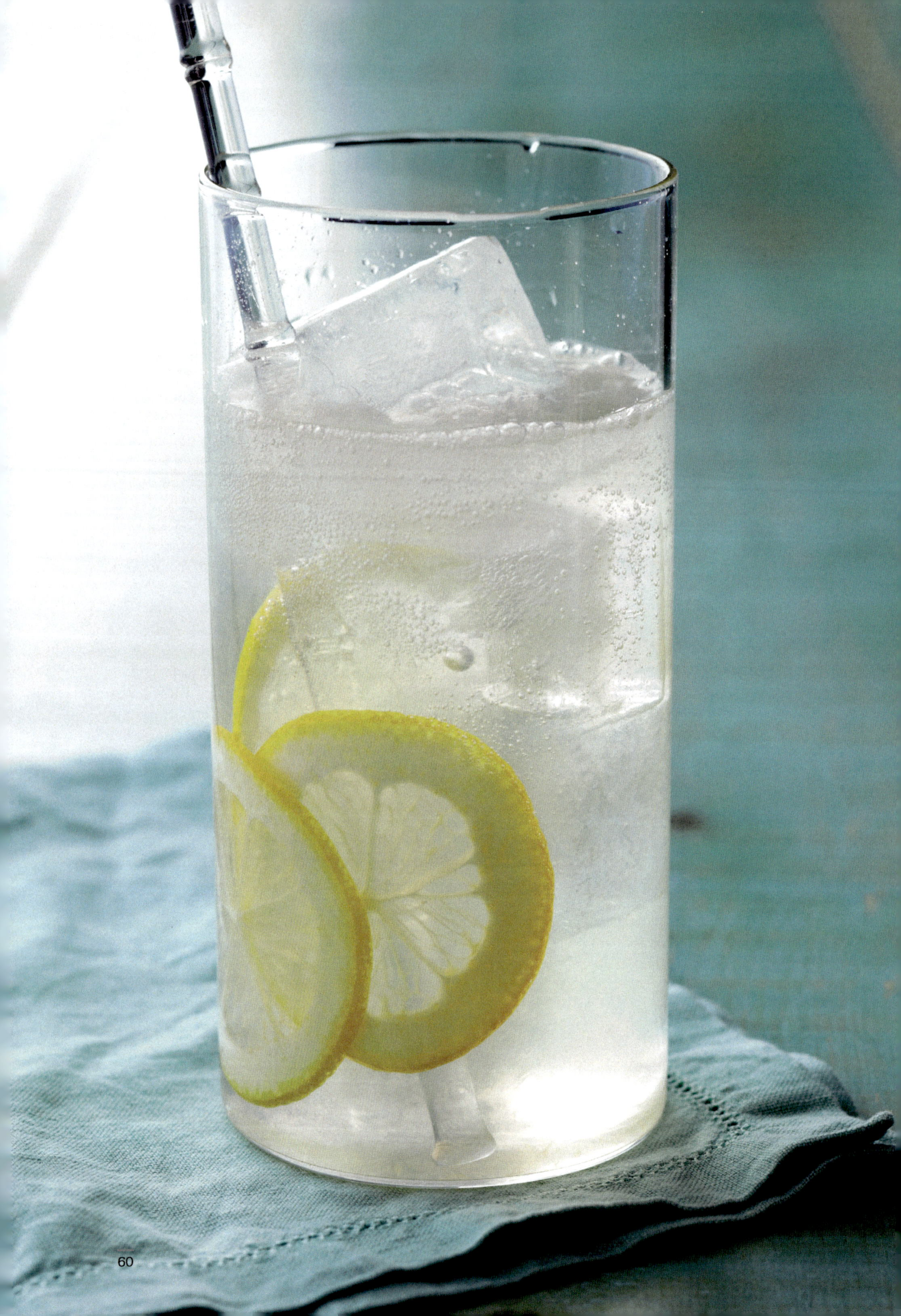

Modern Diet Questions Answered

What are the benefits of lemon water? What about hot yoga? Find out which trends are backed by research

> **By Markham Heid**

YOU ASKED:
Will Drinking Lemon Water Help Me Lose Weight?

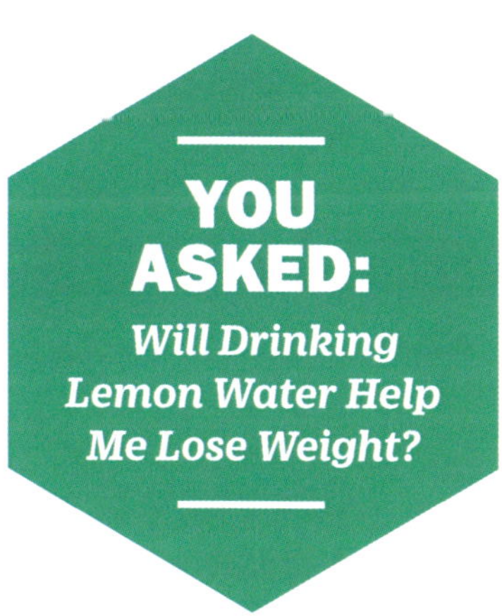

> Lemon-infused water is a popular drink for weight loss. Proponents claim that it flushes out toxins, cuts appetite and tweaks the body's digestive processes in ways that block fat absorption. Trouble is, it doesn't work like that.

The drink's hype seems to stem from a 2008 Japanese study that linked lemons' polyphenols—micronutrients with antioxidant properties—to less weight gain and improved fat metabolism in mice that were fed a high-fat diet. It's possible, the study team said, that lemon polyphenols may stimulate the liver to produce enzymes that help block the absorption of dietary fats.

Keep in mind that the research was in mice; there have been no rigorous studies showing that lemon water can promote weight loss in humans, says Dana Hunnes, a senior dietitian at the University of California, Los Angeles, Medical Center.

Another problem is that lemon water uses the juice, not the rind. Mice in the study were eating a diet loaded with lemon rind, the site of most of the polyphenols in lemons. Many committed lemon-water fans may be zesting some rind into their water, but it's likely nowhere near the amount the mice in the study were consuming.

Of course, lemon is healthy in moderation. It's a good source of vitamin C, and some studies have linked low vitamin-C status to obesity. But that's a large leap from saying that ingesting more vitamin C can prevent or reverse weight gain, Hunnes says.

Pectin, a kind of fiber found in lemons, has also been linked to some weight-loss benefits. "Pectin can lower LDL or bad cholesterol and has some anti-inflammatory benefits," says Bahram Arjmandi, a professor of nutrition at Florida State University and former editor in chief of the *Journal of Food and Nutritional Disorders*. "It can also prevent fat absorption and moderate insulin response." But most pectin comes from the flesh or pith of a fruit, not its juice.

"Lemon water is not a miracle weight-loss food," adds Elizabeth DeJulius, a registered dietitian nutritionist with Alliance Integrative Medicine in Cincinnati. Still, lemon water could indirectly help people lose weight, she says, because thirst is often mistaken for hunger. Because many people find plain water boring, adding lemon may lead them to stay hydrated, reducing thirst-triggered food cravings. "Dehydration can also slow metabolism, which in the long term can lead to weight gain," she says.

Bottom line: If you like lemon water, sip away. But if you're looking for evidence-backed ways to lose weight, this isn't among them.

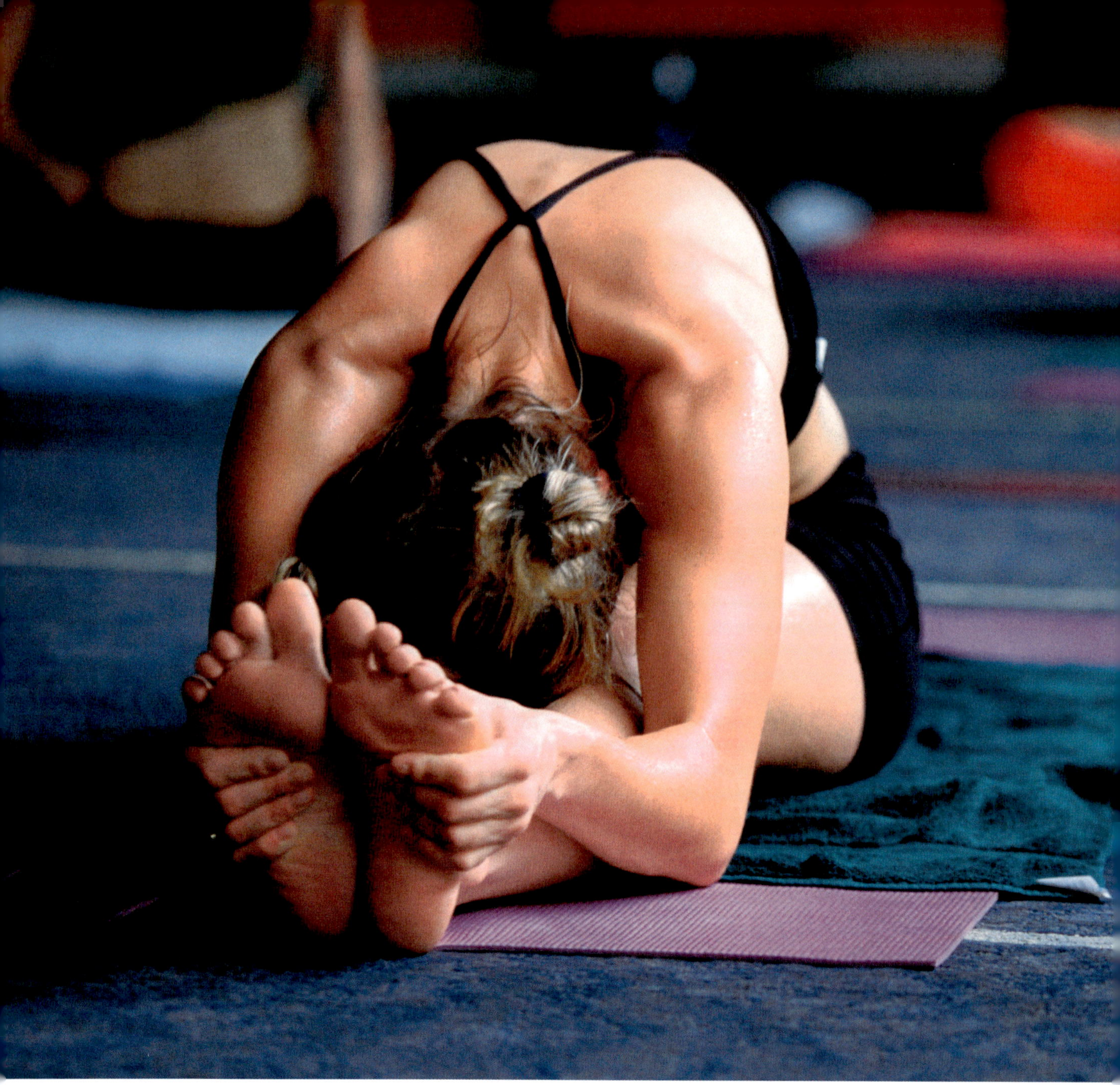

YOU ASKED:
Can You Lose Weight Just from Your Stomach?

> Whether you have extra weight in your upper arms or your rear end, it makes sense that targeting those areas with exercise would slim them down. But in most cases, this kind of "spot reduction" isn't possible. One study in the *Journal of Strength and Conditioning Research* found that six weeks of intensive ab workouts did nothing to slim the exercisers' midsections.

Working out just one part of your body probably won't slim it down, but some body parts, such as your stomach, are more likely to shed fat when you exercise. "Some fat deposits are more metabolically active than others, and those may be more responsive to exercise interventions," says Arthur Weltman, a professor of medicine and chair of the department of kinesiology at the

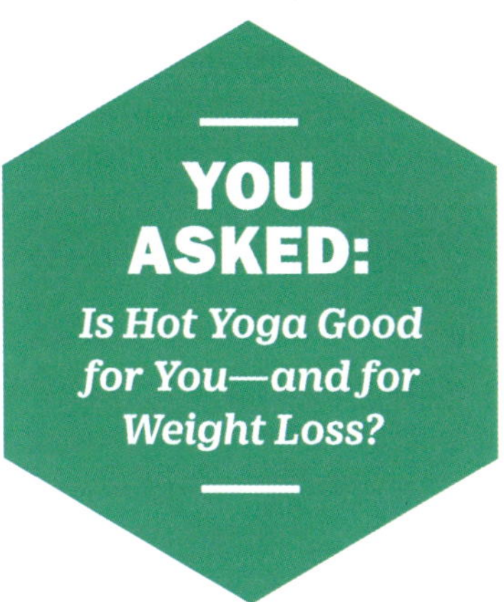

> Start poking around for hard science on Bikram or "hot" yoga and you'll find something curious: there's not much of it. "Considering how popular this is, it's pretty shocking that our study is one of the very first published research efforts on the subject," says Brian L. Tracy, an exercise scientist at Colorado State University.

Tracy and his team have conducted two experiments on the effects of Bikram yoga, which involves completing a series of poses for 90 minutes in a room heated to 104 or 105 degrees. The first experiment included healthy (but sedentary) young adults with no yoga experience. After eight weeks, the participants showed modest increases in strength and muscle control, as well as a big improvement in balance. They also achieved a slight drop in body weight. "To be honest, we were pretty surprised by the small size of the weight change, because when you're in the Bikram studio, you feel like you're working really hard," Tracy says. "And remember, these were people who didn't regularly exercise before the study. We were expecting a bigger drop."

For his follow-up experiment, Tracy hooked up experienced yogis to equipment that measured heart rates, body temperatures and energy expenditures during a typical Bikram session. The new data helped explain some of those disappointing body-weight findings: while heart rates and core temperatures climbed significantly (but not dangerously) during the 90-minute session, the participants' metabolic rates—the amount of calories their bodies burned—were roughly equivalent to those of people walking briskly.

On the other hand, one part of your body is getting a major workout, Tracy says. "Heart rates are quite high for the amount of work you're doing. Quite high."

Is that something you should worry about? "Potentially," says Kim Allan Williams, former president of the American College of Cardiology. When you're hot, your heart pumps large volumes of blood to the vessels in your skin where, through a process called convection, sweat is produced. "And it's actually not the sweat but the sweat's evaporation that helps cool you off," he explains. "Sweat does not evaporate efficiently in those conditions."

The humidity in Bikram studios is supposed to be kept at 40%. But it might be higher. As the humidity climbs and your heart keeps working to cool you off, you're sweating out minerals like potassium and sodium, along with H_2O, Williams says. You may need to replenish lost electrolytes. "It's the same for athletes working out in the middle of summer," he adds. "You have to be mindful of the heat and humidity."

To stay safe, pay close attention to your body. Feelings of light-headedness, nausea, confusion or muscle cramping are warning signs that you need to take a break.

University of Virginia. "Abdominal fat in particular is one of the most metabolically active fats."

Working out triggers the release of hormones, Weltman says. The higher the exercise intensity, the more of these hormones your body pumps out, and the more metabolically active fat you lose.

If you have fat stored in your gut, arms and chest, a lot of your fat is metabolically active, so it will likely respond to exercise and diet changes, he says. The bad news: extra fat in these regions is also linked with a greater risk for diabetes, heart disease and cancer. On the other hand, if you store fat in the hips, butt and thighs, that fat is not metabolically active. You have a lower risk for many diseases, "but that fat is very hard to reduce," he says.

What form of exercise targets the tummy? One study found that while aerobic training—such as running and cycling—led to greater whole-body fat loss, resistance training targeted abdominal fat in particular.

In a nutshell, spot reduction generally doesn't work. But a mix of resistance training and high-intensity aerobic exercise, along with a healthy diet, may help reduce belly fat.

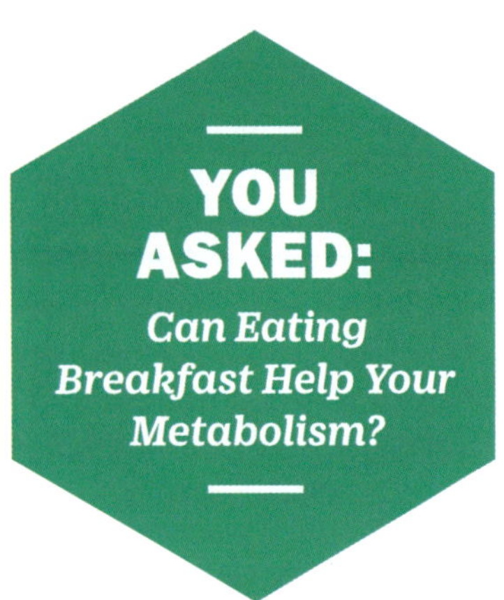

> Plenty of research has found that eating breakfast is important for weight maintenance, metabolism and overall good health. Now, the evidence is even stronger: a small recent randomized controlled trial finds that regularly eating a substantial morning meal directly affects how fat cells function in the body by changing the activity of genes involved in fat metabolism and insulin resistance. The findings suggest that eating breakfast every morning may help lower people's risk for Type 2 diabetes and cardiovascular disease, the study authors say—and that even if a morning meal increases a person's total calorie consumption, those calories may be offset by other energy-burning benefits.

In the study, published in the *Journal of Physiology*, researchers asked 49 people ages 21 to 60 to either eat breakfast or fast until midday every day for six weeks. Those in the breakfast group were asked to eat at least 700 calories by 11 a.m. and at least half of those calories within two hours of waking. They could choose the foods they wanted, but most people opted for typical breakfast foods like cereals, toast and juice.

Before and after the study, the researchers measured everyone's metabolism, body composition and cardiovascular and metabolic health. They also took biopsies of their fat cells to measure the activity of 44 different genes and proteins related to metabolism and other physiological processes, as well as the cells' ability to take up sugar, which is the body's response to changing insulin levels.

They found that in people who had normal weight, eating breakfast decreased the activity of genes involved in fat burning. In other words, there was some evidence that skipping breakfast actually increased fat burning, lead author Javier Gonzalez, an associate professor of nutrition and metabolism at the University of Bath in the U.K., wrote in an email.

But total energy balance—the most important aspect for weight loss or weight maintenance—did not drastically differ between groups. "Breakfast consumption increased total calorie intake in lean people, but this was offset by breakfast also stimulating physical activity energy expenditure in lean people," he wrote.

More important, eating breakfast decreased the activity of genes involved in insulin resistance and increased the amount of sugar the cells took up, which could protect against diabetes. This is "in line with our previous observations that breakfast consumption is associated with better glucose control in fat cells," Gonzalez wrote. "This may have implications for disease risk, but we need to work more on this."

However, that's not what they found in people with obesity. The more body fat a person had, the less their fat cells responded to insulin. At least one gene associated with fat burning was also more active among people with obesity in the group that ate breakfast, compared with the fasting group.

Fasting, meanwhile, seemed to increase the activity of genes associated with inflammation—but only in people with obesity. "Therefore, the guidelines for breakfast consumption should perhaps differ depending on whether people are lean or obese," wrote Gonzalez. More research is needed, he added.

Because the people in the study ate breakfasts high in carbohydrates, the researchers are unable to say whether other types of breakfasts—like high-protein meals—would have the same effects. "However, we are now exploring how different types of breakfast influence health," Gonzalez wrote, "and how breakfast interacts with other health behaviors such as exercise."

The goal is to better understand how fat responds to food at different times of day. "We may be able to uncover new ways to prevent the negative consequences of having a large amount of body fat," Gonzalez wrote, potentially by doing something as simple as eating breakfast daily.

—AMANDA MACMILLAN

In one study, eating breakfast increased the activity of genes involved in insulin resistance, which could protect against diabetes.

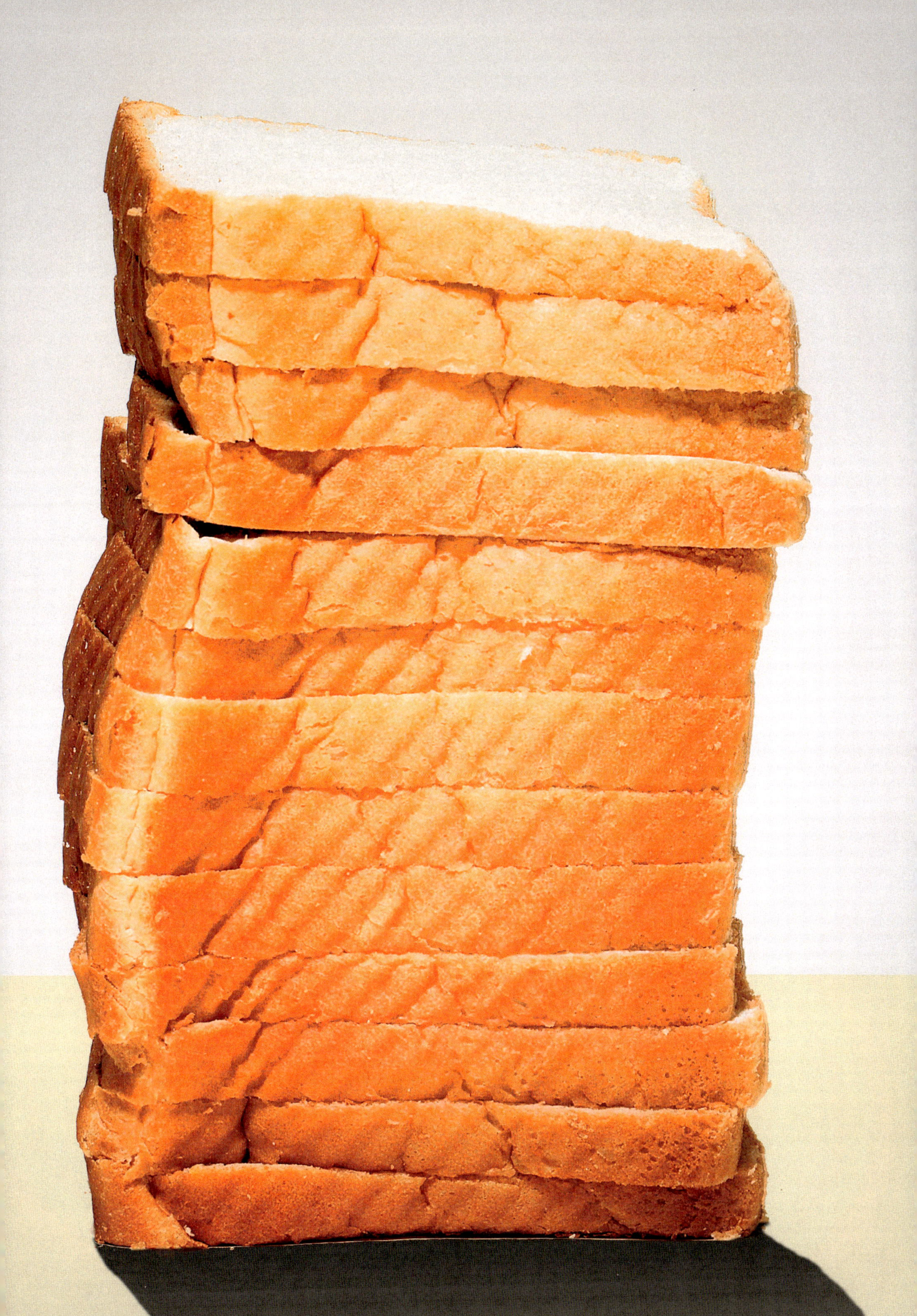

Would You Try Goop's Detox?

Gwyneth Paltrow's plan left our writer inspired to eat healthily—and also hungry

› **By Kathleen Felton**

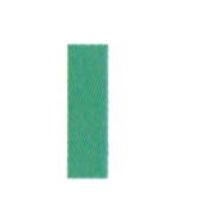

I'M NOT A HUGE FAN OF THE WORD "DETOX." OUR bodies are able to remove toxins on their own naturally, and they don't need additional help from a special diet or juice fast to do so. That said, when Goop (Gwyneth Paltrow's lifestyle website) published its annual detox plan in 2017, I was intrigued. After a holiday diet of cheese plates and sugar cookies, the idea of hitting reset on my healthy-eating habits sounded pretty great. Plus, the plan promises a "lighter, happier, refreshed you"—sold.

I wasn't thrilled by the idea of feeling hungry for five straight days, but two other things scared me even more than that. First, this plan requires a lot of meal prep. Second, coffee. I average two to three cups a day, and going cold turkey sounded like torture, especially when I thought about the proven health benefits of coffee we'd be giving up. So I compromised: I made all of Goop's recipes except for the lunches, since it would be easy to instead buy meals with detox-approved ingredients. I cut back my coffee intake, rather than totally eliminate it.

I walked away from the five days feeling energized, inspired to eat more healthily—and very, very hungry. Here's exactly how it went.

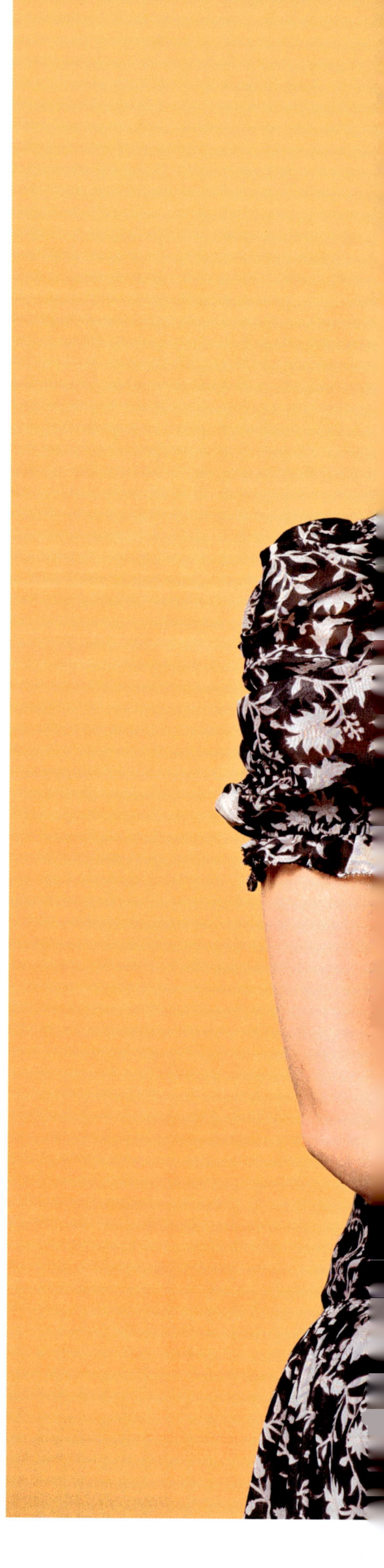

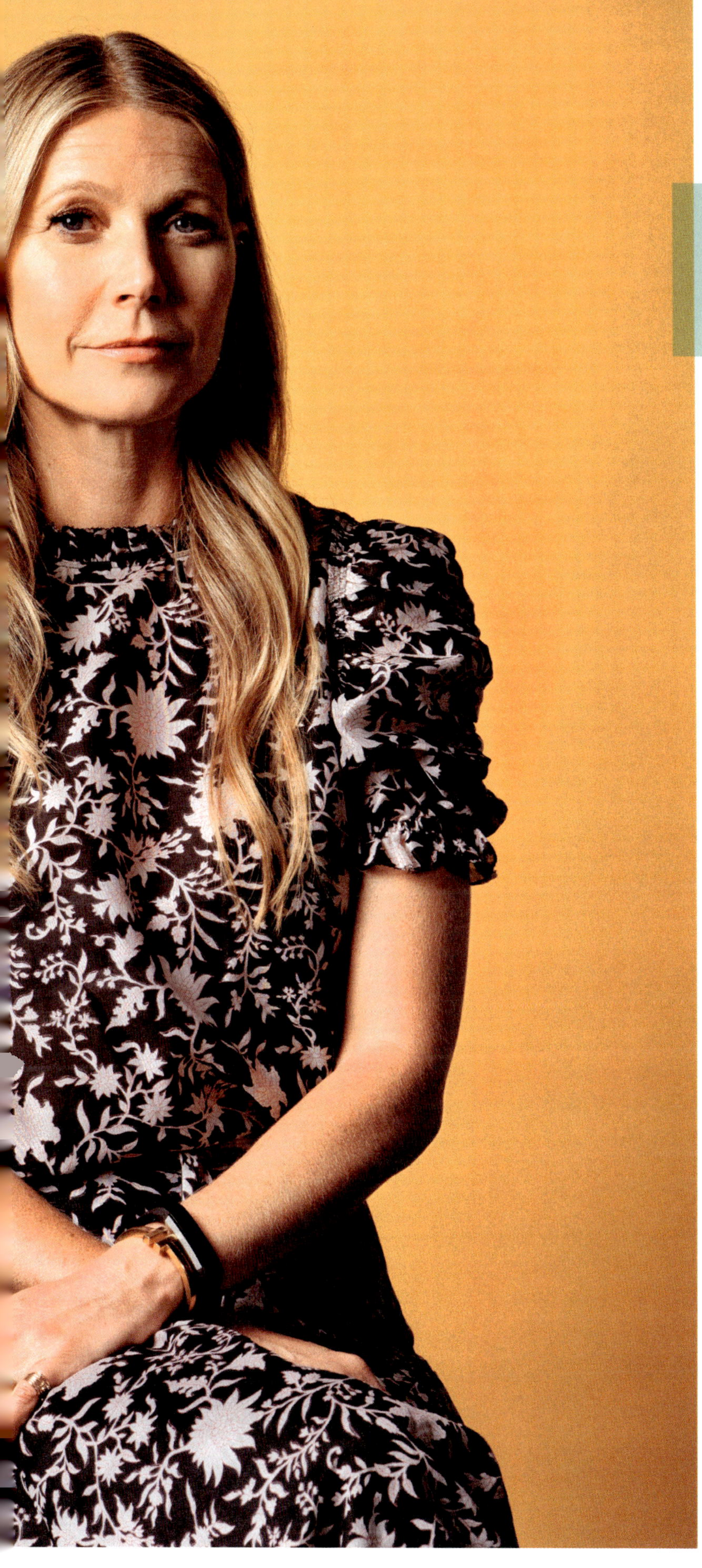

Gwyneth Paltrow's lifestyle brand, Goop, is reportedly worth $250 million.

Day 1: Sunday

My detox did not get off to the best start. I woke up on Sunday morning, forgot I had agreed to do this and promptly had two cups of espresso. (It had been a late Saturday night—sorry, GP.)

I'd stocked up on most of the detox supplies earlier in the week, but I had a few things left to buy. So I went to my local health-food store to spend an upsetting amount of money on almonds, pumpkin seeds, sunflower butter and coconut nectar. (For the uninitiated, coconut nectar is like a more expensive and less delicious cousin of honey.) After that, it was time to bake Gwyneth's Detox Granola Bars—the recipe for which is found, along with many others, at goop.com. Those bars would be my breakfast for the next five days.

They were easy enough to make: you use a blender to turn the walnuts and gluten-free oats into a fine, flour-like powder, and then combine all the ingredients in a bowl and spread the mixture onto a sheet pan. The result? While flavorful, they were the most dry and crumbly granola bars in the entire world (I don't think I will ever fully decrumb my kitchen). But at least I could feel good about snacking on them—with almonds, flax seeds, walnuts and pumpkin seeds, they deliver a serious dose of protein and healthy fats.

Next up: Gwyneth's Warming Morning Latte, which I decided to make even though it was technically the afternoon. The latte calls for 13 different ingredients, including sunflower butter, coconut nectar, coconut oil and "transformational" powders from a brand called Sun Potion that retail for a cool $125 altogether. I love my job, but dropping that much money on dubious powders seemed above and beyond the call of duty. I tried to call in press samples from the company, but they didn't come, so I made the latte with the other 10 ingredients.

It was actually kind of good. While definitely not a coffee replacement, the drink was creamy and foamy at the top, thanks to coconut oil. And with spices like ground nutmeg, cloves and cinnamon, it tasted Christmassy and a little nutty.

Dinner was Lentils with Salmon and Grilled Radicchio, which turned out to be my least favorite of all the recipes. The salmon and lentils were fine, but I'm not a fan of bitter greens, and grilled radicchio is extremely bitter, even with balsamic vinegar on top.

How is Goop food? The veggie salad with poached chicken (top) was a hit; the salmon and radicchio, a miss.

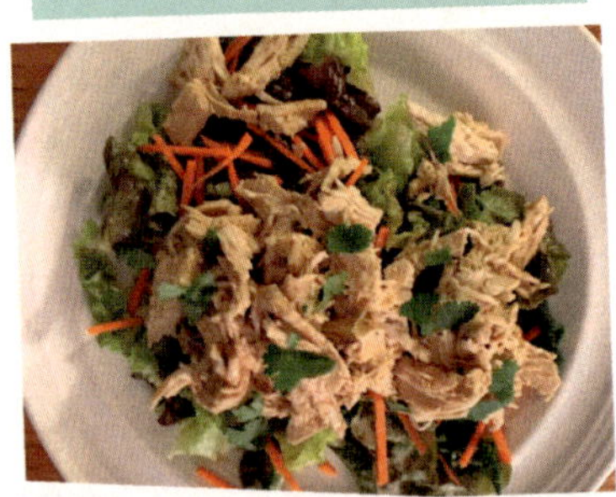

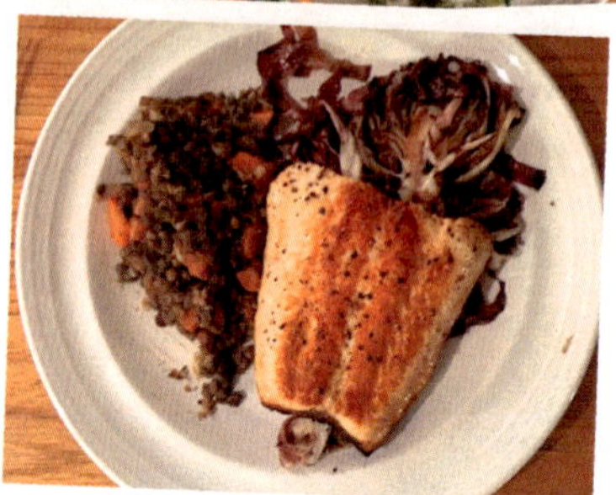

Day 2: Monday

Breakfast: crumbly granola bar and two well-intentioned cups of hot lemon water before I caved and had a coffee. Lunch: salad from the company cafeteria with romaine lettuce, carrots, chickpeas, cucumbers, sunflower seeds and tuna. I usually have a mid-afternoon snack of Goldfish or M&Ms (they're free in my office, so hard to resist), but since they're not Goop-approved, I had an apple. Meh.

By the end of the workday, I was starving, so I decided I'd make the Turkey and Sweet Potato Chili for dinner, which seemed like the heartiest of the recipes. And also did I mention I was starving? The chili was awesome, and the recipe makes a *ton* of it. My red-meat-loving fiancé (now my husband), whom I somehow convinced to do this with me, even said he'd have this for dinner again.

Day 3: Tuesday

Another dry granola bar for breakfast and some dry brown-rice sushi for lunch (the detox does not allow soy sauce, which I sometimes forget is the tastiest part of sushi). I had one cup of coffee, which, while still cheating, was a huge improvement from my usual two to three cups.

For dinner, I made the Laarb Lettuce Cups. I liked them a lot, but the last chicken lettuce cups I had were from Chrissy Teigen's cookbook, so this was a lesson in contrasts. The sauce in Gwyneth's version is a lot less flavorful than Chrissy's (which benefits from lots of sriracha, hoisin and Thai sweet chili sauce), but I admittedly felt a lot lighter after these.

Maybe too light—I was still hungry after dinner, so I had another granola bar and made myself a warming latte. It was good, but ugh, is it a pain to measure out all the different spices just for one little drink.

Day 4: Wednesday

I went with a granola bar for breakfast (they were starting to grow on me a little bit) and the leftover chili from day two for lunch. I'd gone to yoga class on Sunday and Tuesday, but this was going to be my first cardio workout of the week, and I was curious to see how much energy I would have for it. I was able to complete seven out of the eight circuits—not bad.

For dinner, I made the Crunchy Veggie Salad with Poached Chicken and Garlicky Sunbutter Dressing, which was my second-favorite recipe after the chili. If there's anything Gwyneth knows well, it's aromatics: the chicken is cooked with cilantro stalks, shallot, garlic and ginger, and it was way more flavorful than any other poached chicken I'd ever made. I also became obsessed with the garlicky sunbutter dressing, which tastes like very creamy peanut sauce.

And some exciting news: the Sun Potions arrived! The three that Gwyneth recommends for the warming latte are Sun Potion astragalus, Sun Potion tocos and Sun Potion reishi. Since they cost $125 altogether, I wanted to believe that these powders would basically change my life. But not having any idea what they actually were, I asked Cynthia Sass, RD, for her professional opinion before giving them a try. "There's some research to show that rice bran may help lower cholesterol," she said of the tocos. "It provides soluble fiber, so it may boost fullness." She added that there's also some scientific research to suggest that astralagus might improve athletic performance and regulate blood glucose and insulin levels in people with Type 2 diabetes.

But Sass scared me away from the reishi: "It's thought to boost immunity and reduce inflammation," she said, but there was a fatal case of fulminant hepatitis when powdered reishi mushroom was taken orally for longer than one month. "It can also interact or interfere with some medications."

Yeah, nope. I left the reishi at my desk and took home the toros and the astralagus for my evening warming latte. I did feel like the powders bulked up the drink a bit, making it more filling and protein-shake-like. But I'm not sure there was a big difference in taste. (In other words, save your $125.)

GP's chili (bottom) was tasty and satisfying, but the lettuce cups were blah and didn't satiate our fearless detoxer.

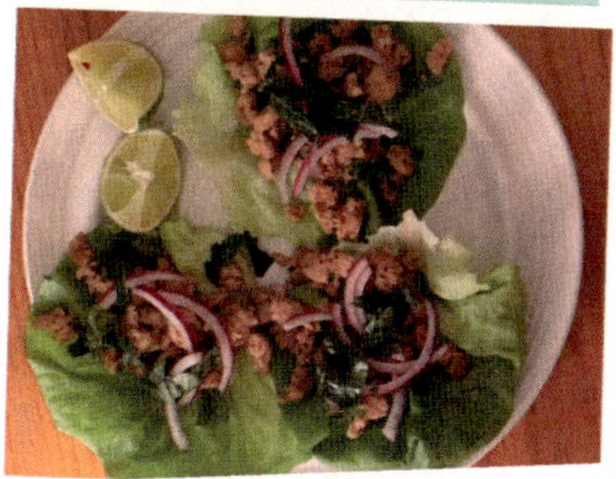

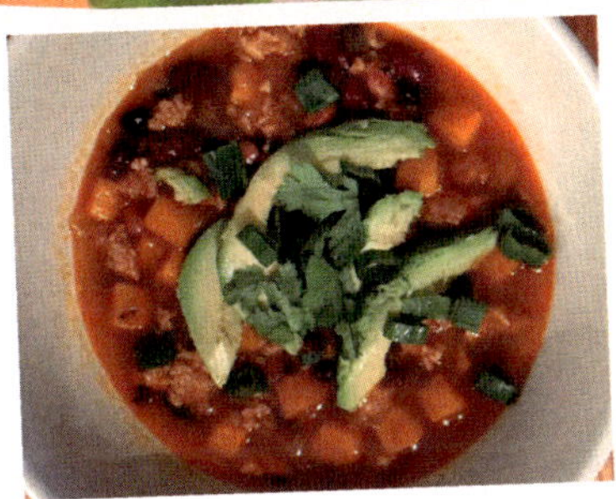

Day 5: Thursday

I skipped breakfast (bad, I know) and had a salad for lunch with greens, avocado, sunflower seeds, cucumber, Kalamata olives and chickpeas, and an apple with peanut butter for my afternoon snack. I don't think there was enough protein in my salad, because I left work the hungriest I've ever been. Dinner was the Kitchen Sink Thai Fried Rice, which I was really looking forward to because—rice! Carbs, I have missed you so much. I like the concept because you throw in all the remaining veggies you had to buy for the detox so they don't go to waste. I was so hungry, I forgot to take a picture before eating it. It was really good, but maybe a bit lacking in protein.

Final thoughts

It is now Friday morning and I am very hungry. I can't wait to have two cups of guilt-free coffee today, a sandwich for lunch and pasta for dinner. I weighed myself this morning, and I've lost five pounds on this detox, which seems like a lot in such a short amount of time, especially since I wasn't overweight to begin with.

But I do feel as if I have had more energy than usual, even as I have cut back on caffeine. And temporarily eliminating sugar and dairy was a good exercise—I admittedly probably consume more of these food groups than is ideal, and giving them up forced me to load up on healthier substitutions (for example, adding avocado to my salads instead of my go-to feta). I also like that I've been eating tons of leafy greens, and the recipes got me to try veggies I don't usually reach for at the supermarket, like bok choy.

These past five days have also made me realize that even though I consider myself to be a healthy eater, I rely a bit too heavily on carbs to create a filling meal. I also snack on the free Goldfish and M&Ms in my office more often than I've previously admitted to myself. Going forward, I'll try to eat fewer refined carbs and less red meat and sugar (too much sugar and red meat can increase the risk of heart disease). But I'll be happily adding back whole grains (a good source of filling fiber), shellfish (clams are packed with vitamin B12) and soy. I'm sorry, GP, but I just can't have a sushi roll without soy sauce. □

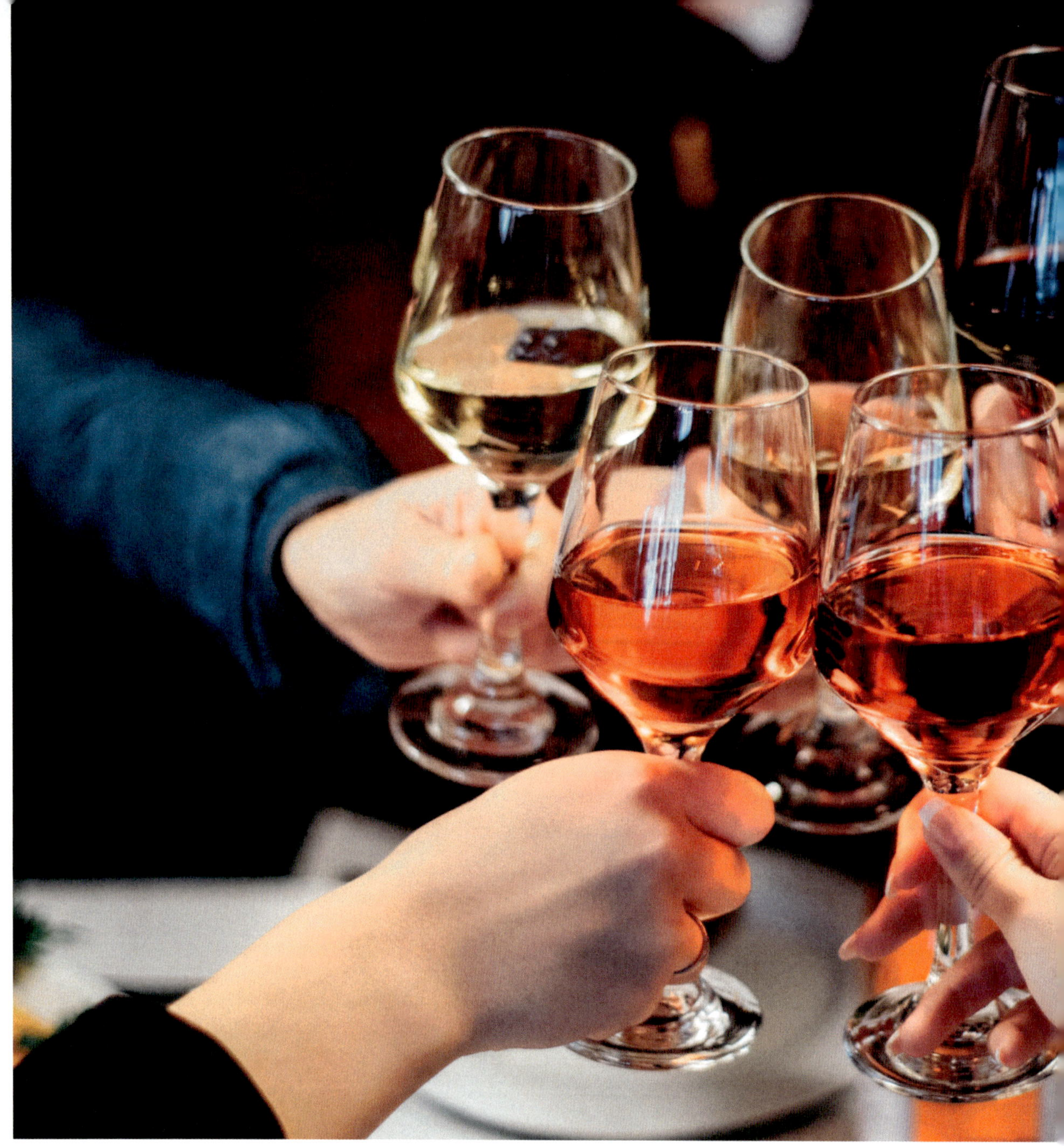

Wine vs. Your Waistline

Beer, wine and other booze don't have to lead to weight gain. Read this before your next night out to avoid cocktail calories

> ***By Sunny Sea Gold***

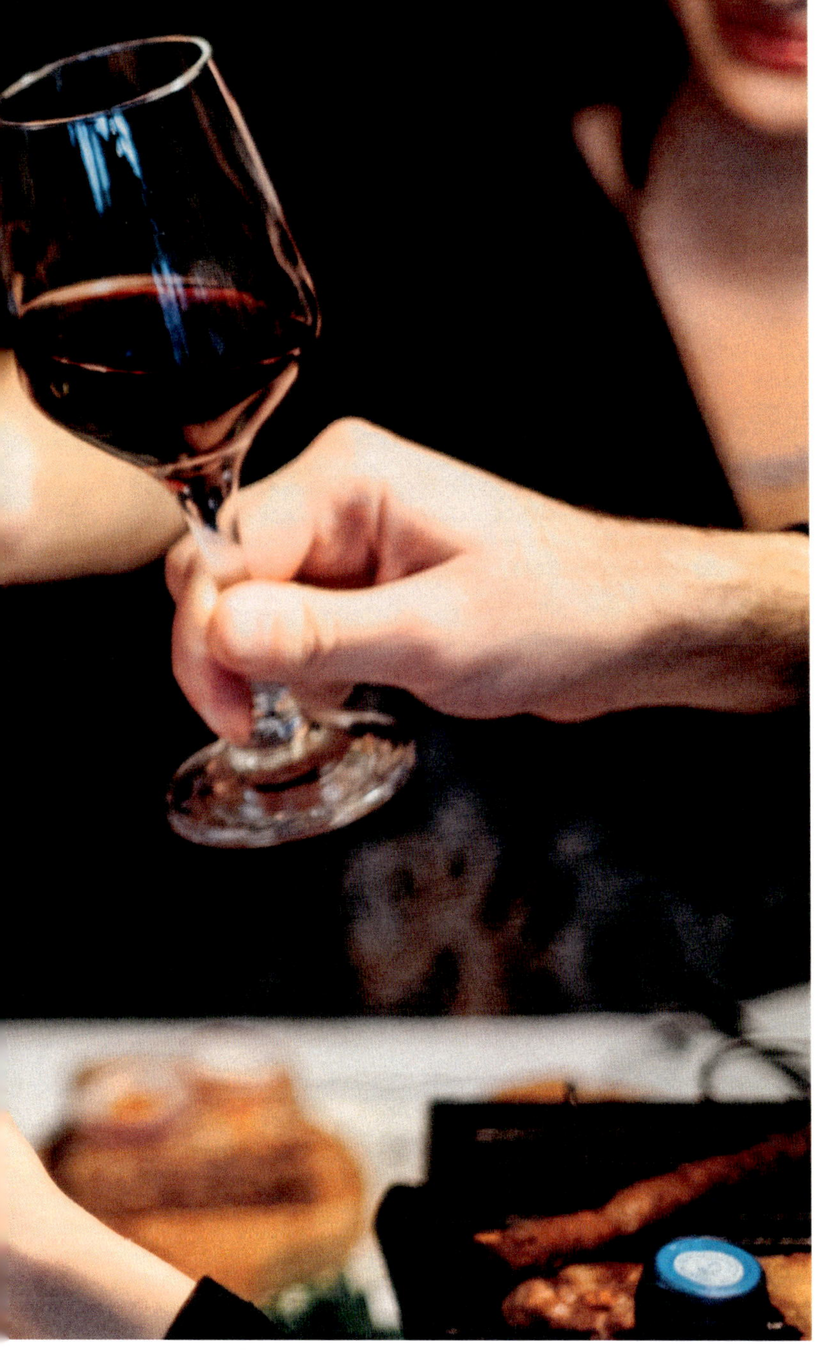

LET'S FACE IT: SOMETIMES THERE'S NOTHING BETter at the end of a long day than a glass of wine. But sipping much more than that can wreak havoc with your shape, and not just by adding hundreds of calories to your diet. Alcohol temporarily keeps your body from burning fat, explains integrative-medicine specialist Pamela Peeke, author of *The Hunger Fix*. Your body can't store calories from alcohol for later, the way it does with food calories. So when you drink, your metabolic system must stop what it's doing (like, say, burning off calories from your last meal) to get rid of the booze.

"Drinking presses 'pause' on your metabolism, shoves away the other calories and says, 'Break me down first!' " Peeke explains. The result is that whatever you recently ate gets stored as fat. What's worse: "Research has uncovered that alcohol especially decreases fat burn in the belly," Peeke adds. "That's why you never hear about 'beer hips'; you hear about a 'beer belly.' "

So can you ever enjoy a drink without putting on pounds? Absolutely, if you do it the right way. In fact, large, long-term studies published in the *Archives of Internal Medicine* and the *International Journal of Obesity* found that middle-aged and older women who drank moderately (about one drink a day) gained less weight over time than those who never imbibed at all; they were also less likely to become obese.

It's a complex topic, but JoAnn Manson, a professor of medicine at Harvard Medical School and co-author of the studies, says that the moderate drinkers appeared to be more likely to compensate for the occasional drinks by taking in fewer calories from other sources and also tended to be a little more physically active. (In other words, they didn't get blitzed on margaritas and then dive into a bowl of fried ice cream.) What else beyond basic exercise and watching what you eat can keep happy hour from turning into hefty hour? Here is how you can fit booze into your healthy-shape plan.

Rule #1: Always eat when you drink

Although the Harvard research suggests it's wise to factor in those cocktail calories, it's actually more important to eat right than to eat less, the experts stress. Skimping on food in order to "make room" for drinks will only backfire and send you straight to the bottom of the candied-nut bowl. Here's why: most cocktails are loaded with simple carbohydrates, "so during a night of drinking, people end up with soaring blood sugar, followed by a 'crash' that leaves them ravenous," says Jason Burke, an anesthesiologist and hangover researcher who runs a hangover-treatment clinic in (where else?) Las Vegas.

You can help counteract that effect by nibbling foods that provide long-lasting energy. "Before you go out, have dinner or a snack with protein, fiber and healthy fat," says Karlene Karst, author of *The Full-Fat Solution*. "They stabilize your blood-sugar levels without slowing down your metabolism." Karst recommends Greek yogurt with berries, almond or hemp butter with an apple, or a protein shake. An added benefit of grabbing a bite beforehand, she says, is that that Pinot or appletini will be absorbed more slowly into the bloodstream, minimizing its diet-damaging effects.

In addition to revving your appetite, tippling also makes you lose your eating inhibitions ("I only live once. I'll have the fettuccine Alfredo!"). "It temporarily impairs the prefrontal cortex, the smarty-pants part of the brain that allows you to think clearly and rein in impulsivity," Peeke says. "So after a certain amount of alcohol—and it's different for everyone—you're going to feel yourself not caring and letting it rip with food and probably drinks." A cocktail (or three) can make you forgetful too, as in, forgetting that the Death by Chocolate dessert is not on your eating plan.

The trick is to have an easy-to-follow strategy in place before you take that first sip. Scout out the bar or restaurant menu ahead of time and note your picks on your phone. Then set an alert to remind you to order wisely—that way you won't have to think too much (or rely on that alcohol-impaired prefrontal cortex!) to stay on track. As with your pre-partying meal, go for something with fiber, protein and a little bit of healthy fat to help control blood-sugar levels and make you feel satisfied, Karst says.

Rule #2: Know that some drinks make you hungrier than others

When it comes to waist-friendly cocktails, the simpler the drink, the better. Not only do the sweet-and-fancy ones tend to have more calories, but the additional sugar can make you even hungrier: your blood sugar skyrockets higher than it does on beer, wine or a shot of something, making the plummet (and the resulting cravings) worse.

And then there are the calories! Booze has seven calories per gram, making it the second-most calorie-dense macronutrient. (That's just below pure fat, which has nine calories per gram.) This means a measly 1.5-ounce jigger of vodka has almost 100 calories. Mix that up with some club soda and lime, and it's a reasonable tipple, but when you start tossing together a whole bunch of different liquors, whether it's a hipster fizz made with bourbon, elderflower liqueur and house-made bitters, or a dive-bar Long Island iced tea loaded with vodka, rum, tequila and gin, it really adds up (to the tune of 300 calories, in the case of a Long Island).

Even simple mixed drinks like rum-and-Cokes and screwdrivers pack extra calories because of the sugary soda and juice. "So if you're going to drink, have something straight up and simple like wine or beer," Peeke advises. Any wine or beer works, but to trim about 10 calories per glass, choose a rosé or white wine instead of a heavier red. A whole pint of a dark beer is about 170 calories (compared with 195 for the same amount of regular beer) and may leave you feeling fuller than, say, champagne, because it's so starchy and rich, Karst notes. Vodka, gin or bourbon with club soda and a twist are pretty good bets too. Club soda is calorie- and sugar-free and dilutes the alcohol and its effect on your cravings. Avoid juices, liqueurs (which are sweet and syrupy), colas, tonics and super-sugary bottled mixes like the ones for a lot of bar-made margaritas and daiquiris.

Rule #3: Stick to a drink or two, tops

No more than one drink a day for women and two a day for men is the widely accepted definition of moderate drinking, but there's a misconception among some bar-hoppers that you can go without alcohol all week and save your seven drinks for the weekend. "That's the worst thing you can possibly do for your weight," Peeke says. (And, of course, for your health.) "It has a much bigger effect than one drink a day."

When you down three or four drinks in one night, your body has many hundreds of alcohol calories to process before it can continue to break down food calories or stored fat. Plus, all those drinks throw

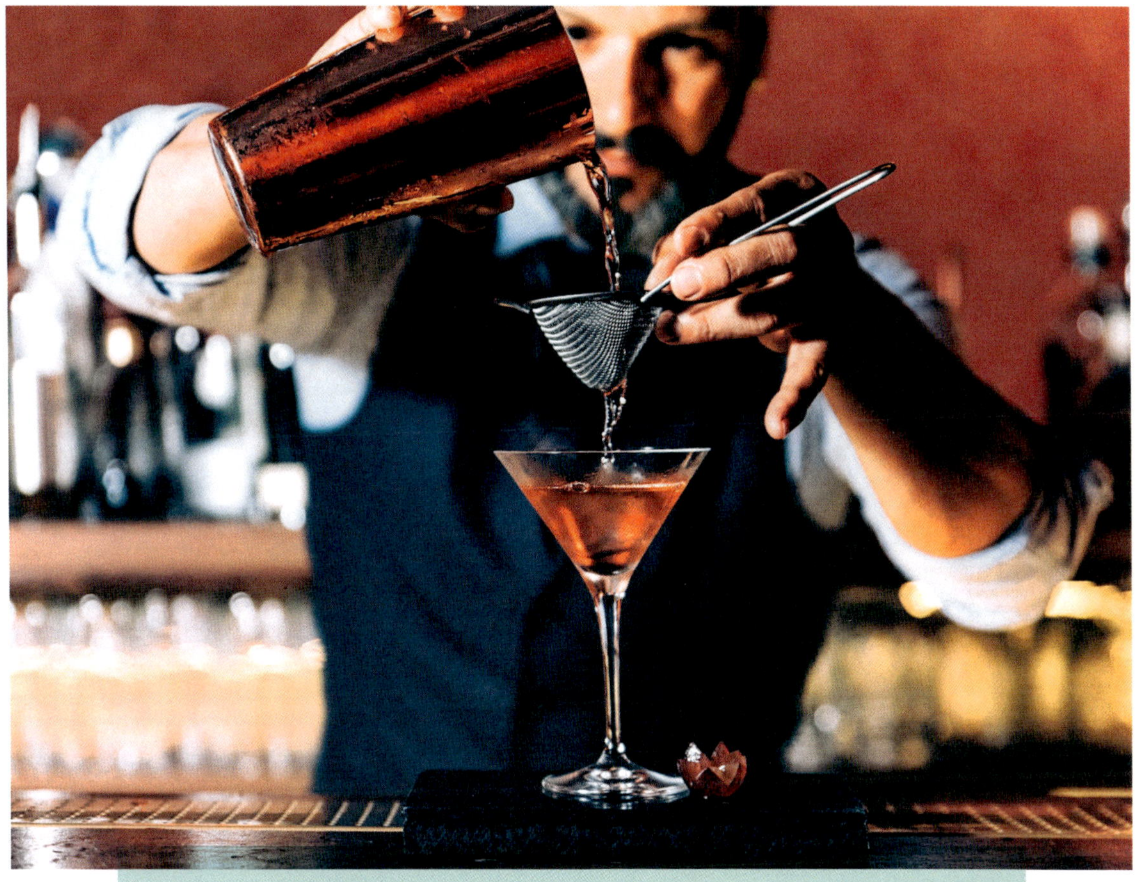

Signature cocktails are fun every now and then, but they often have a lot of sugar and calories; you're better off making beer or wine your go-to drink.

your blood sugar even more out of whack, so you're hungry as heck, and because you're tipsy, your prefrontal cortex is misfiring and you now have zero compunction about ordering the fried mozzarella sticks with a side of ranch (and keeping them all for yourself). The extra calories alone are enough to pile on the pounds; have four drinks every Saturday night and you'll be up about 10 pounds in a year.

Rule #4: Beware that gnawing, starving feeling the next day

The morning after poses a new challenge. As if a hangover weren't punishment enough, you're fighting cravings for large amounts of cheesy, greasy fast food. Part of the problem is that you're dehydrated (don't forget, alcohol is a diuretic), and that can make you feel even hungrier, Karst notes. But that's not the only thing at play. "The body needs energy to resolve the effects of a big night of drinking, so it wants the richest source of energy it can find, which is fat," Burke says. "Also, greasy foods tend to settle the stomach a bit."

To avoid that problem: When you're out, make sure you drink a big glass of water for every cocktail you have. Then, before going to bed, have some more water, along with a snack that is high in fiber and protein such as high-fiber cereal or oatmeal, Burke recommends. "You'll get important nutrients into the body that were lost during alcohol consumption," he explains. "Plus, foods rich in fiber stay in the stomach longer, so you'll be less prone to hunger in the morning."

With any luck, you'll also be less likely to overeat in the a.m., ensuring that your shape won't have to pay a steep price for a fun night out. □

Chapter 3

Power of EXER

Test your fitness level, build abdominal strength,

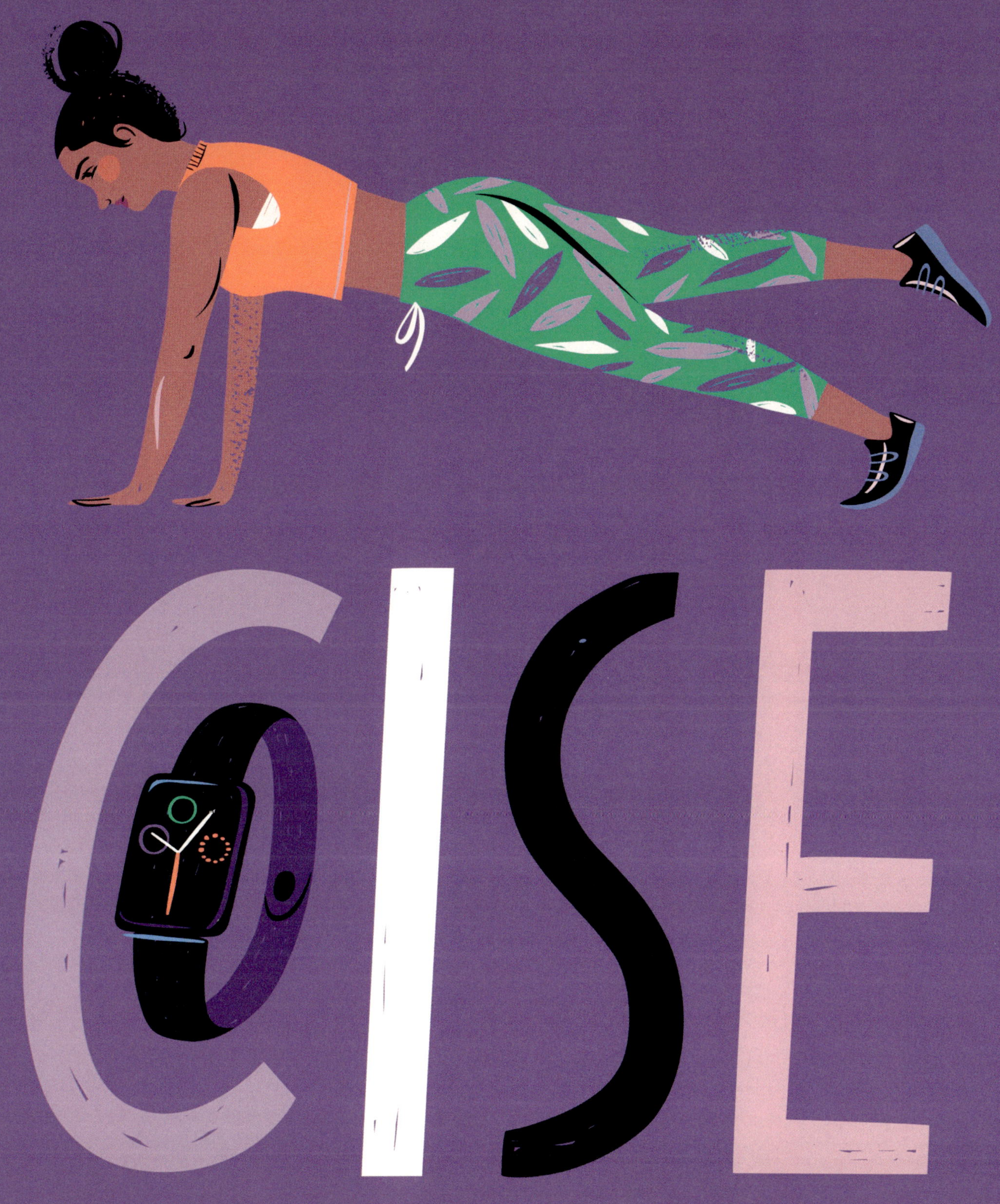

stay motivated and make walking a super workout

How Fit Are You?

Take these at-home tests to measure your cardio, strength, flexibility and balance. Then use our easy steps to improve your scores

> ***By Natalie Gingerich Mackenzie***

ON YOUR MORNING JOG, YOU CAN'T HELP BUT NOTICE every time another runner blows past you. During yoga, you know it's not zen to compare yourself, but you wonder how your neighbor to the right gets into those shapes.

Sound familiar? We all want to know how we measure up—and that's actually a good thing. "Exercisers do better when they test—and retest—themselves," says Kevin Asuncion, a National Academy of Sports Medicine–certified personal trainer. "Feedback motivates you when it's positive and helps redirect your efforts when it's not."

It's not just about winning your age group in the local 5K fun run, either. Having an honest benchmark of your own fitness level gives you a concrete number to beat—essential for setting S.M.A.R.T. (specific, measurable, actionable, relevant and time-bound) goals. That's why it's a good idea to regularly assess your cardio power, strength, flexibility and balance: four pillars of physical fitness. Put yourself to the test, then use the strategies on these pages to improve your score on any (or all!) fronts.

Are you aerobically fit?

> How to find out: Walk a mile

Not everyone is a runner, nor do you need to be in order to be fit. But if you can walk a mile, you can estimate your VO2 max, the measure of how efficiently your body uses oxygen. This is important

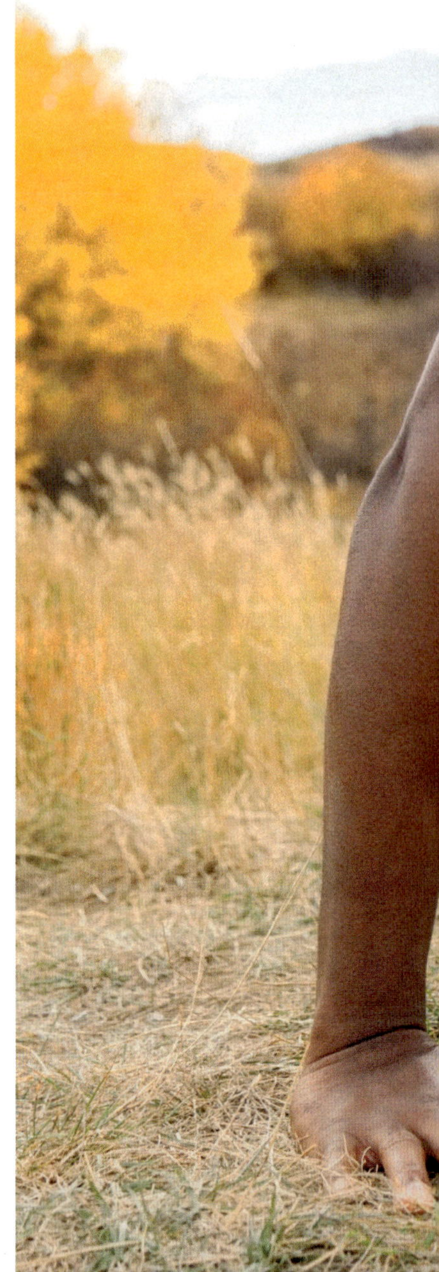

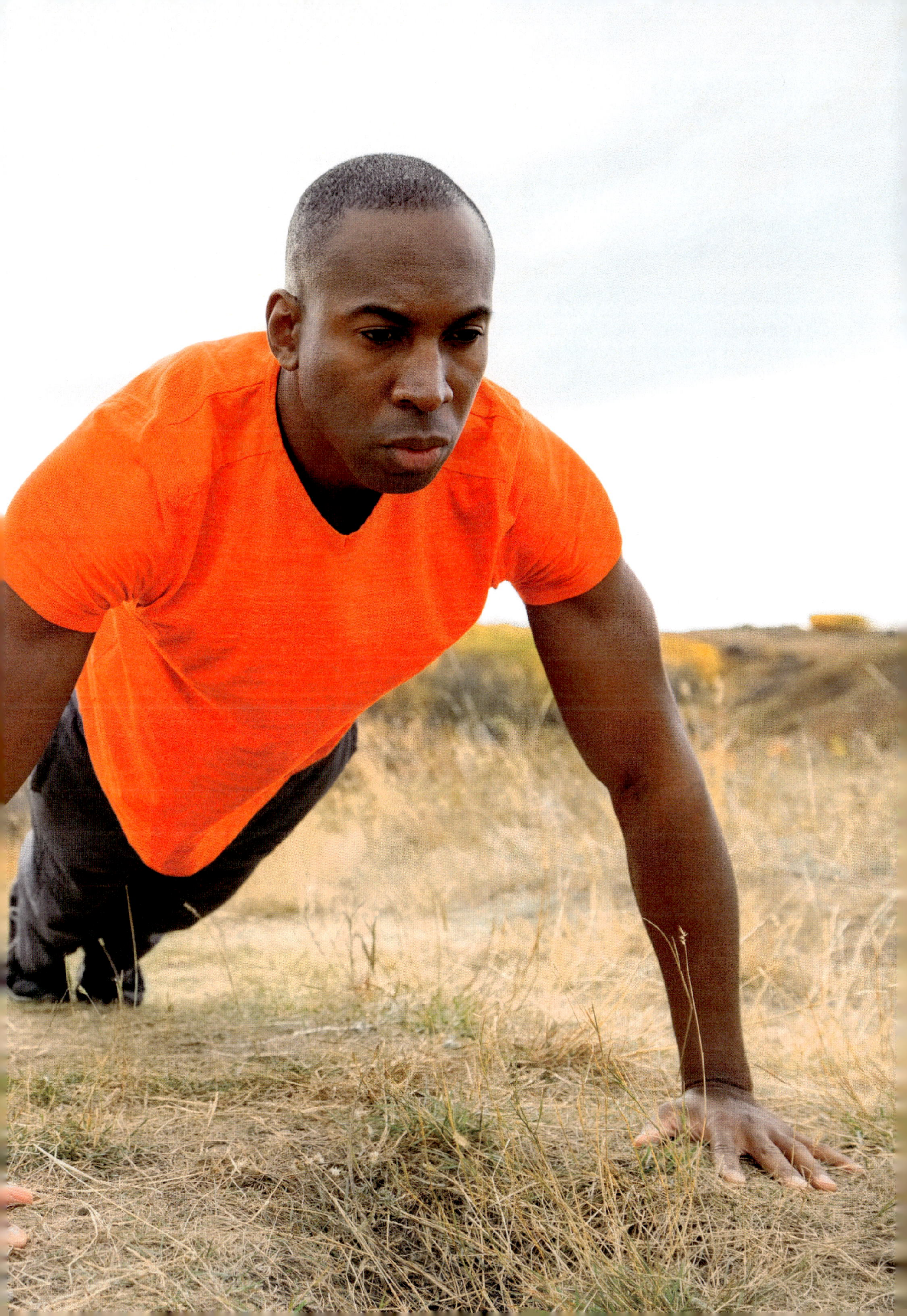

because studies suggest that, whatever your weight, higher levels of aerobic fitness may be protective against health conditions like diabetes and even early death from all causes.

> **Try it.** Head to a track or use your car's odometer to measure out a (flat) one-mile course. Walk the distance as fast as you can, timing yourself with a stopwatch. As soon as you finish, check your pulse. If you have a heart-rate-monitor watch, you're set. If you don't, DIY by feeling for it on your wrist. Count the beats for 10 seconds and multiply by six to get your beats per minute.

> **Score it.** Search online for the Rockport Walk Test calculator and plug in your gender, age, weight, time for the mile walk and your heart rate at the end. Or calculate it yourself with this formula: 132.853 – (0.0769 × weight in pounds) –(0.3877 × age) + (6.315 × 1 if you're male or 0 if you're female) – (3.2649 × time in minutes) – (0.1565 × heart rate).

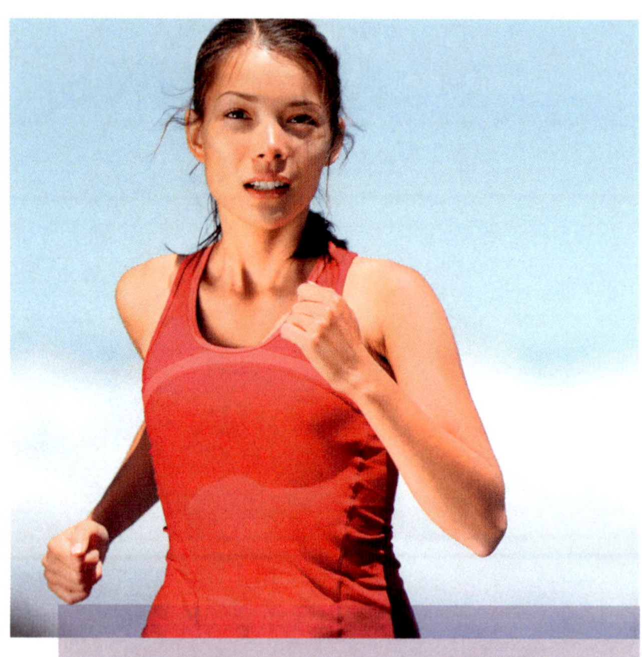

Mix intervals (higher-intensity bursts) into your cardio to boost cardiovascular fitness.

A score of around 40 is good for men in their 30s and 40s. Forty-eight or higher, and you're a stud. For women in their 30s, 37 or above is good. Female and over 40? Aim for 33 or higher. A number of 40 or above is exceptional.

> **Get faster.** To improve your score, add intervals—short bursts of higher-intensity effort—to your cardio sessions. Since they push your heart and lungs to work harder than they're used to, they deliver faster results than if you were to continue at your regular pace. "We used to think intervals were only for the super fit because they're so difficult, but they can benefit everybody," says Michael Ross, medical director of the Rothman Orthopaedic Institute's Performance Lab in Bryn Mawr, Pa.

And you can reap the rewards of intervals with the cardio of your choice (running, biking, etc.). After warming up at a conversational pace, pick it up to a level where it's hard to get a full sentence out for one to two minutes. Slow down to recover for two to three minutes and then repeat, aiming for 20 to 30 minutes total.

As you get fitter, Ross recommends incorporating intervals in a variety of speeds and durations to challenge all of your muscle fibers. That means short and fast efforts of just 20 to 30 seconds all-out as well as longer intervals of 8 to 10 minutes at a pace you can just maintain for that amount of time (followed by a recovery period).

Are you strong?

> **How to find out: See how many push-ups and squats you can do**

While the truest measure of strength is the greatest amount of weight you can lift with any given muscle group, those tests can be grueling—and risky. Instead, try testing your muscle endurance on two key exercises, the push-up and the squat, suggests Chris Gagliardi, a trainer, coach and medical-exercise specialist who teaches fitness professionals with the American Council on Exercise.

> **Try it.**

1. Push-up test. Get into a plank position with your elbows bent and hands planted below your shoulders. Men should extend their legs, supporting themselves on their hands and toes, body in a straight line from the head to the heels. Women should do a modified push-up on hands and knees. Keeping abs tight, straighten your elbows to press up. Repeat and count how many you can do until you can't go any longer.

2. Squat test. Stand with your feet hips width apart, toes pointing forward. Keeping weight on your heels, bend your knees and sit back. Aim to lower until your thighs are parallel with the ground, keeping knees behind toes. Push into heels to stand. Count how many reps you can do until you need to rest.

> **Score it.** For push-ups, 13 to 19 is a solid count for women in their 30s. For 30-something men, 17 to 21 is a good score. For the squat test, about 30 is a good number to hit for women ages 36 to 45, while men that age should aim for a count in the upper 30s. If you're up to a decade older than that, subtract five from your goal number. Younger? Add five.

> **Get stronger.** The recipe for getting stronger is to create what's called "overload" by regularly challenging your muscles to do slightly more than they're used to. You can do this by using weights, resistance bands or body-weight exercises (like push-ups and squats) two to three times a week. (Do it only once a week and you may find you feel sore after every session.) Shoot for 8 to 12 reps of each exercise.

While practicing squats and push-ups is a solid start, to make sure you hit all your major muscle groups, you should include moves that involve pushing, pulling, squatting and twisting, says Ross. Another hint: exercises that use just one arm or leg at a time tend to be most effective, he says.

Are you flexible?

> **How to find out: Check your hips and hamstrings**

Since the hips and hamstrings link the upper and lower body, they're a good gauge of general flexibility. The tests here are preferable to the classic sit-and-reach, which can aggravate back pain, says Jessica Matthews, an assistant professor of kinesiology at Point Loma Nazarene University and the author of *Stretching to Stay Young*.

> **Try it.** Lie faceup on an exercise table or bench, your lower legs hanging off the end. Bend right leg and pull knee toward your chest. Next, lie fully on the table with both legs extended; lift right leg toward the ceiling without bending your knee. Do both tests on each side.

> **Score it.** On the first test, if you can pull your knee to about chest level without lifting your opposite leg and lower back off the surface, your hip flexibility is good. Ditto on the second test, if you can lift your leg to 80 degrees. Less than that means you've got tight hamstrings, which can tug on your lower back, pulling your posture out of whack and causing pain.

> **Get more flexible.** Lie faceup in doorway, left knee bent and right hip near right side of door frame. Extend right leg to the ceiling, back of leg against the edge of the door frame. Flex foot, pressing heel toward the ceiling. Hold for 20 to 30 seconds. Repeat on left leg. Do up to three times a day.

How's your balance?

> **How to find out: Do the Romberg test**

Balance may be the easiest component of fitness to ignore while you're young. It's the unsung hero that keeps you from wiping out when you step on a patch of ice and helps you stay upright on a moving bus. A well-tuned connection between your body's sense of space and your muscles firing is essential to every move you make, from walking to running to standing on your tiptoes to reach the top shelf.

"If you have a sedentary job or life, you may not even realize you have a balance issue until it's too late or a fall happens," says Gagliardi of the American Council on Exercise.

And it's not just about preventing falls. Research shows that not only is poor balance a risk factor for musculoskeletal injuries like ankle sprains, but also, training your balance could actually make positive changes in your brain to improve memory and spatial reasoning.

> **Try it.** Stand near a wall with your feet together, arches touching, and cross your arms in front of your chest. Set a timer and close your eyes. The goal: stand this way without wavering or falling for one minute. If you can do that, you've got a good baseline for balance. Overachiever? Try the sharpened Romberg test: stand with your feet in line heel to toe, eyes closed.

> **Score it.** If you can do the sharpened Romberg test for 60 seconds, it's a good sign, says Gagliardi.

> **Get better balance.** Practice the Romberg test. Go to the level that feels safe for you, even if that's sitting on the edge of a chair with your feet together; aim for three 30-second holds. Progress to standing with a narrow stance. If you ace the test, incorporate balance into your strength training with one-legged exercises like lunges or by turning two-legged exercises (like a bridge) into one-legged ones (extend one leg). □

Secrets from Star Trainers

Even celebrities need help with motivation. Tap this advice from Hollywood's top fitness pros to bust past any plateau

> **By Myatt Murphy**

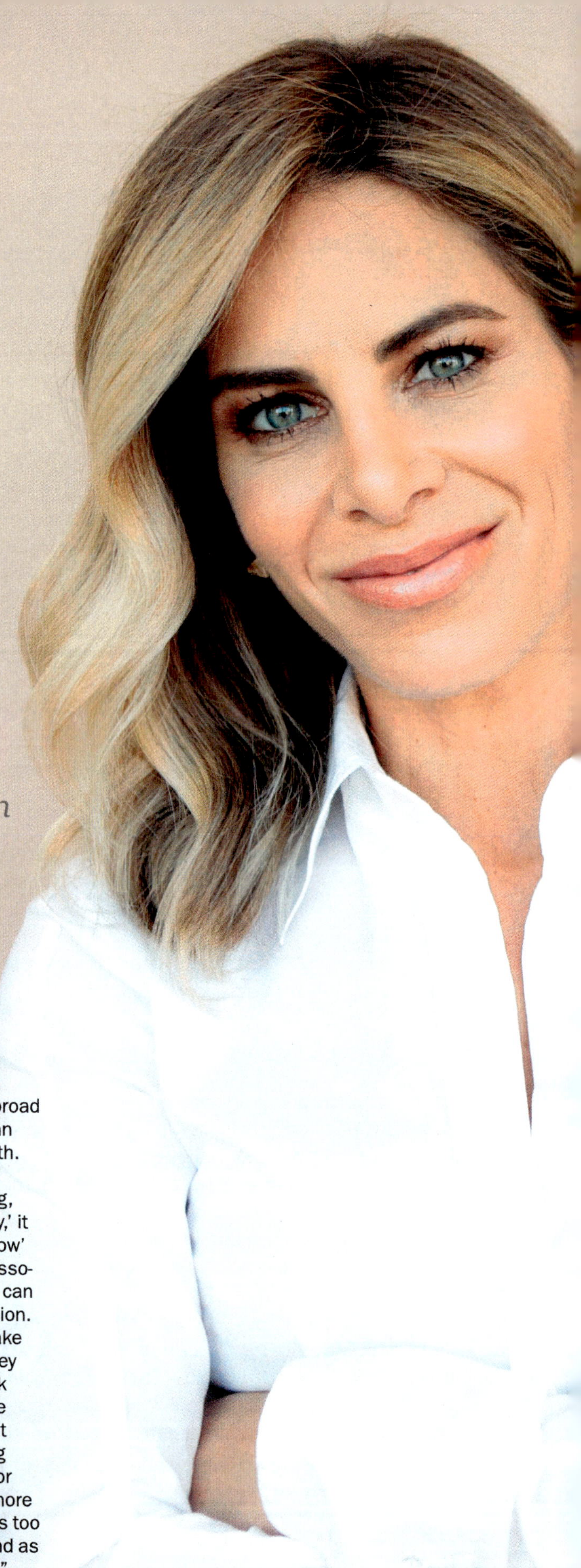

"Remind yourself of your 'why'"

—Jillian Michaels, *personal trainer and eight-time* New York Times *best-selling author (her latest book is* The 6 Keys*)*

"Nothing in life worth having comes easy or for free, be it a healthy relationship, a healthy career or, in the case of fitness, a healthy body. But when I ask people why they work out, most think in generalities, saying they do it 'for their health' or 'to look better.' But that's like saying you want to travel northeast—it's way too broad and impossible to form an emotional connection with. Exercising without a purpose in mind is punishing, but when you have a 'why,' it helps you tolerate the 'how' (the work and sacrifice associated with the goal) and can turn exercise into a passion. I tell everyone to really take time to consider 'why' they want to be healthy or look better—and how their life will improve as a result. It could be for your wedding day, being a role model for your kids or just having more confidence—no reason is too superficial or too profound as long as it matters to you."

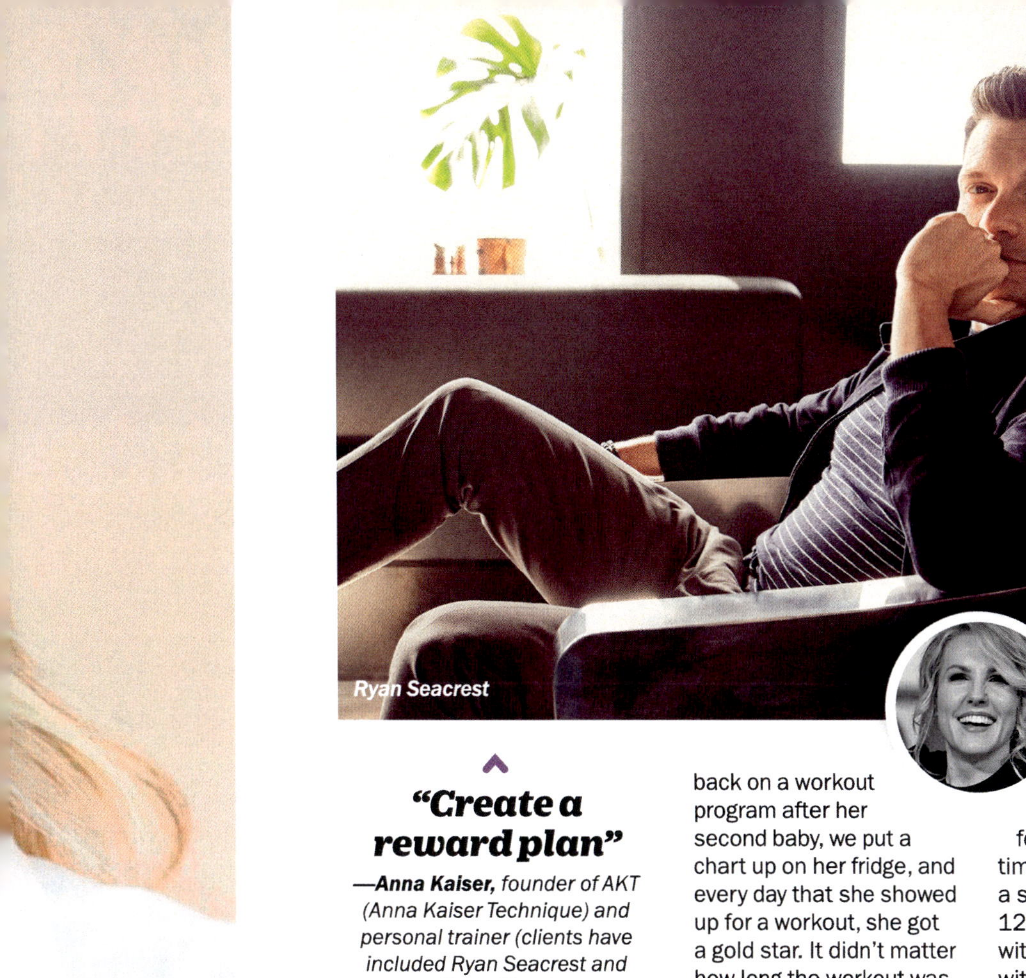

Ryan Seacrest

"Create a reward plan"

—**Anna Kaiser,** *founder of AKT (Anna Kaiser Technique) and personal trainer (clients have included Ryan Seacrest and Karlie Kloss)*

"When I was getting Shakira back on a workout program after her second baby, we put a chart up on her fridge, and every day that she showed up for a workout, she got a gold star. It didn't matter how long the workout was. Whether you exercise for 5 minutes, 10 minutes or an hour, every minute counts—just aim for three days a week for one month. Every time you do, give yourself a star, and when you reach 12 stars, reward yourself with a manicure or lunch with a friend. It's all about re-committing and creating a new habit, which makes exercise much easier!"

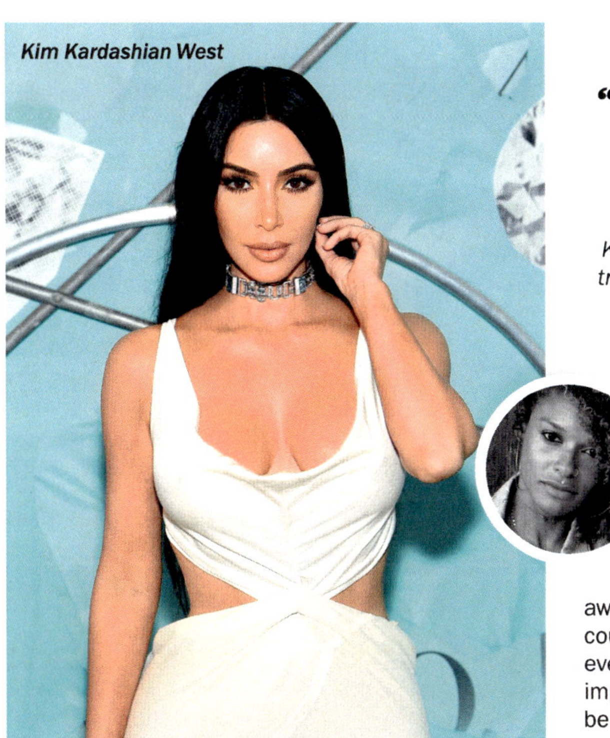

Kim Kardashian West

"Think about how every muscle is moving"

—**Melissa Alcantara,** *Kim Kardashian West's personal trainer and creator of the 8-Week Body Sculptor program*

"It's quality, not quantity, that gets the best results at the gym. No matter what exercise you perform, stay completely aware of your body and how it moves from head to toe. S-L-O-W down and bring deep awareness to your breath. By not counting, but focusing on making every movement feel like the most important thing you ever did, you'll be more excited about exercise and yield the best results."

"Find your flaws—and steer toward them"

***—Stephen Pasterino,** Victoria's Secret models' go-to trainer (clients include Nadine Leopold, Devon Windsor and Blanca Padilla), and creator of the low-impact method P.volve*

"Most people love to do only workouts they're good at, which can cause a repetitiveness that causes many to plateau (that is, hitting a state of little or no change). Instead, try figuring out what you're *not* good at, and then make it your goal to conquer those types of exercises, workouts or machines—or at least get better at doing them. You'll find yourself recharged by feeling a sense of competition with yourself, and you'll also end up training your body in ways that can take you to new heights of health."

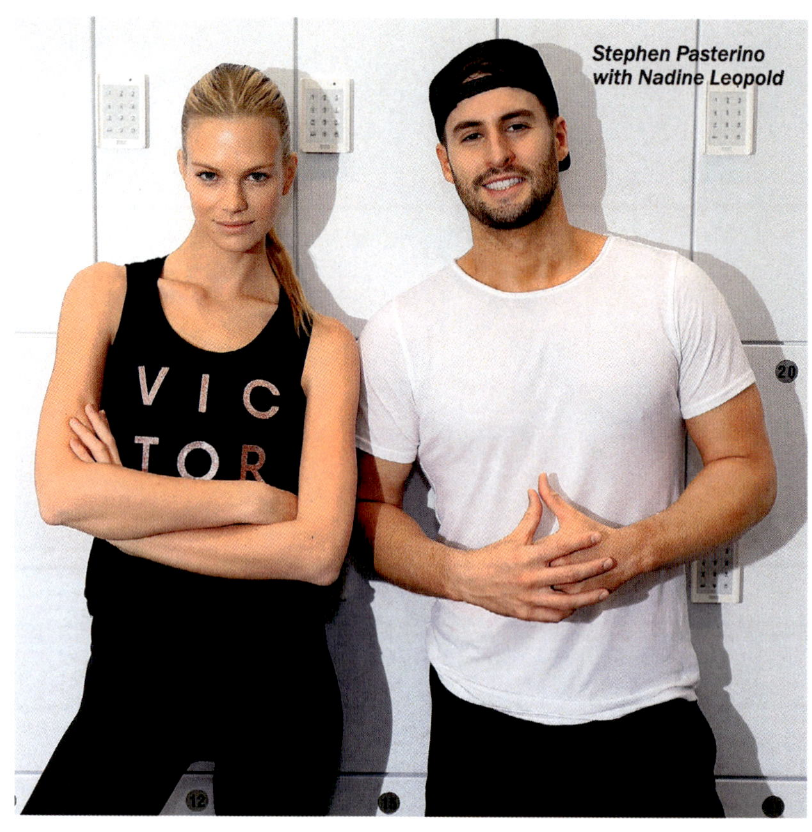

Stephen Pasterino with Nadine Leopold

Ryan Reynolds

"Change things up well before you check out"

***—Don Saladino,** celebrity trainer whose clients include Ryan Reynolds, Blake Lively and Scarlett Johansson; owner of Drive495; and creator of the Playbook exercise app*

"Everyone waits until they're bored with workouts before they mix things up. That's a mistake that can cause you to stop working out. Instead, switch up your program a week before you normally get bored (usually after three to six weeks). You're doing it right if you're continuing to see results but it's just beginning to feel like you're going through the motions. Just don't switch them up every session; that will keep you from seeing results that can be motivating."

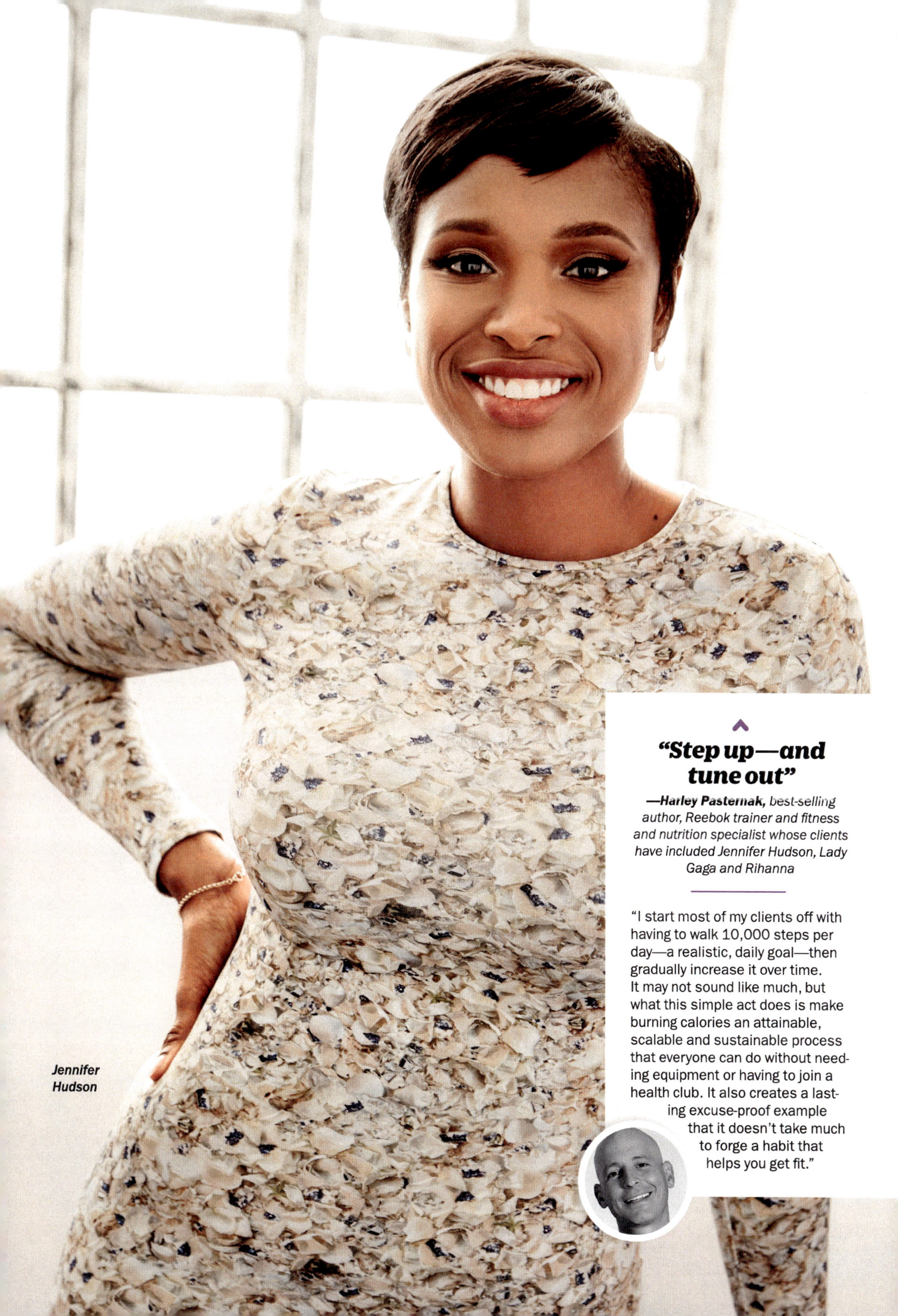

Jennifer Hudson

"Step up—and tune out"

***—Harley Pasternak,** best-selling author, Reebok trainer and fitness and nutrition specialist whose clients have included Jennifer Hudson, Lady Gaga and Rihanna*

"I start most of my clients off with having to walk 10,000 steps per day—a realistic, daily goal—then gradually increase it over time. It may not sound like much, but what this simple act does is make burning calories an attainable, scalable and sustainable process that everyone can do without needing equipment or having to join a health club. It also creates a lasting excuse-proof example that it doesn't take much to forge a habit that helps you get fit."

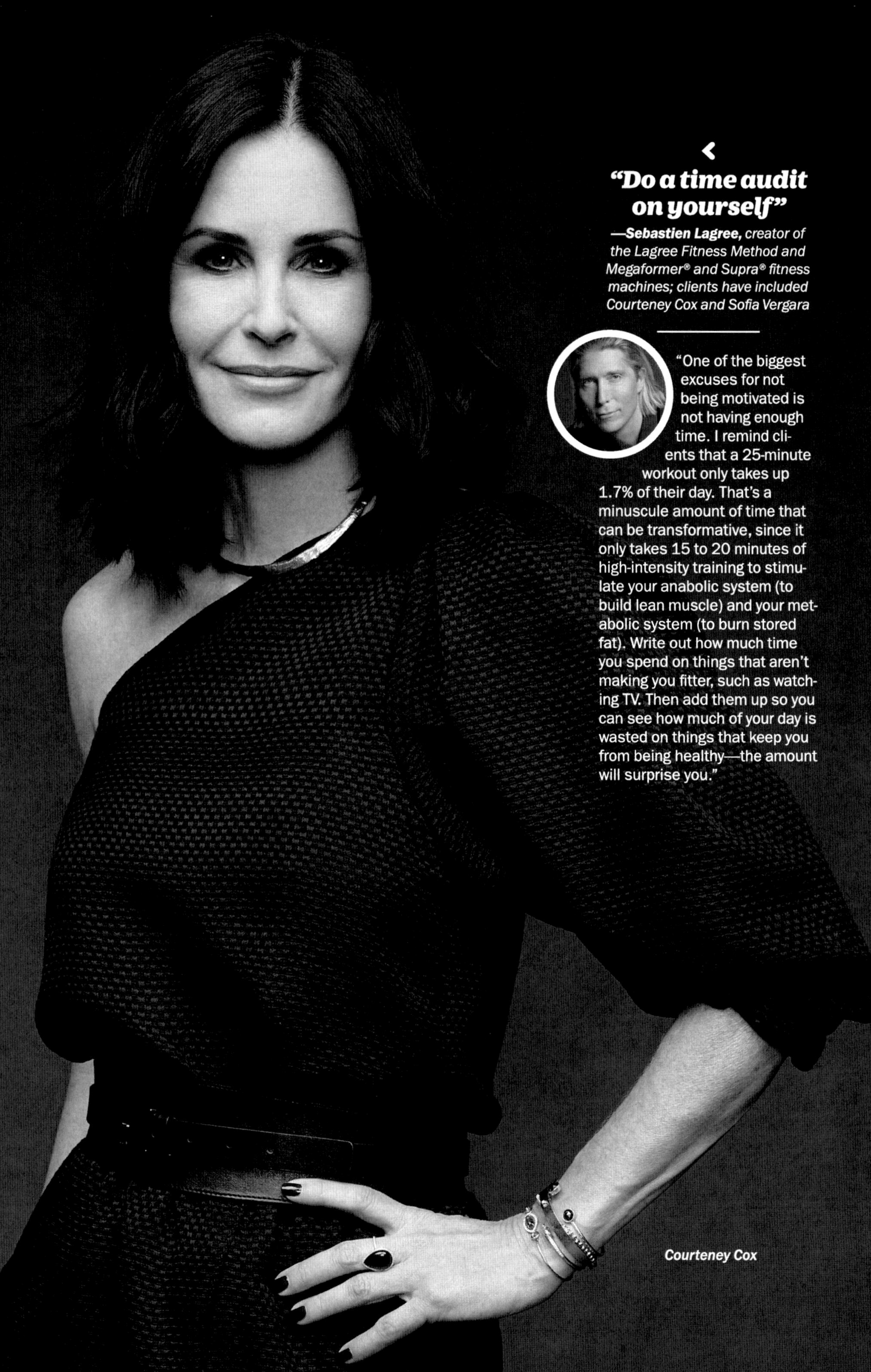

“Do a time audit on yourself”

—**Sebastien Lagree,** *creator of the Lagree Fitness Method and Megaformer® and Supra® fitness machines; clients have included Courteney Cox and Sofia Vergara*

“One of the biggest excuses for not being motivated is not having enough time. I remind clients that a 25-minute workout only takes up 1.7% of their day. That’s a minuscule amount of time that can be transformative, since it only takes 15 to 20 minutes of high-intensity training to stimulate your anabolic system (to build lean muscle) and your metabolic system (to burn stored fat). Write out how much time you spend on things that aren’t making you fitter, such as watching TV. Then add them up so you can see how much of your day is wasted on things that keep you from being healthy—the amount will surprise you.”

Courteney Cox

"Learn to wait and you'll look great"

—**Shaun T,** *creator of Insanity, Beachbody and Transform: 20; Missy Elliott and Cher have done his program*

"The biggest mistake people make is putting too much pressure to achieve a fitness goal by a certain date. Instead, think about getting in shape as making a series of small changes and winning little victories. Did you take the stairs instead of the elevator, or replace your diet soda for water? Then count those as milestones. Before you know it, all of those small wins will turn into a big victory of feeling better, having more energy and being on the authentic path to a happier, healthier life!"

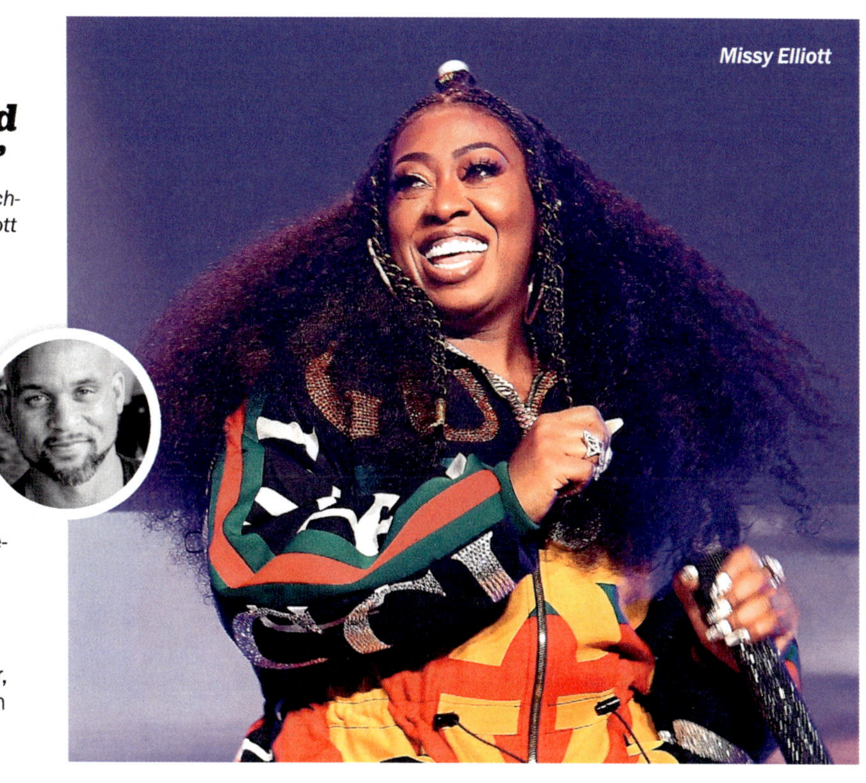

Missy Elliott

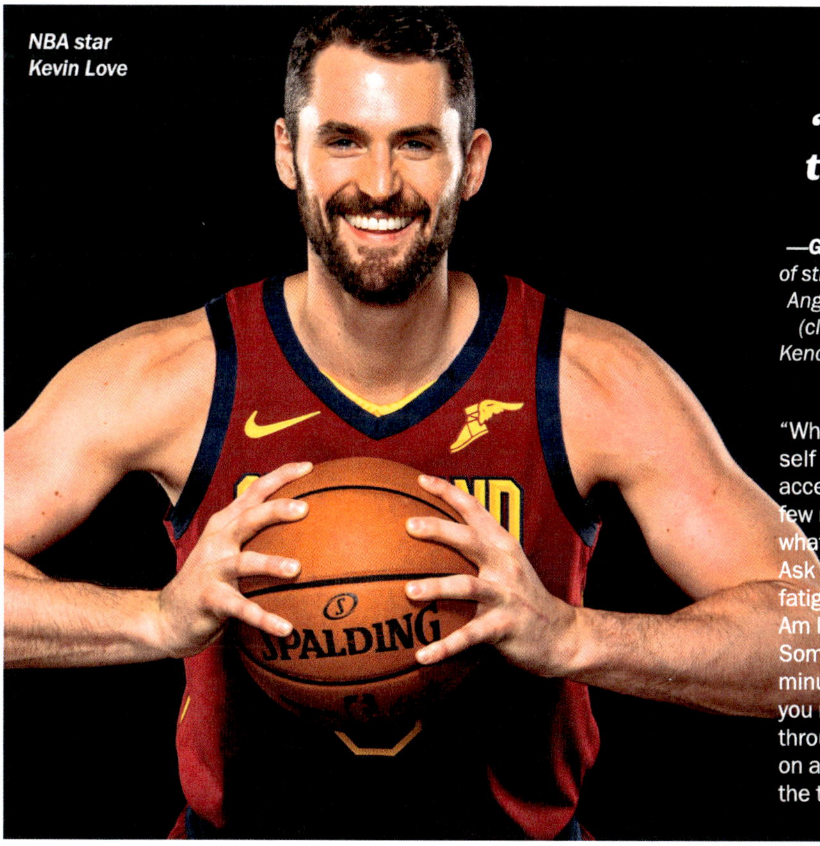

NBA star Kevin Love

"Use your brain to outthink your body"

—**Gunnar Peterson,** *author, director of strength and endurance for the Los Angeles Lakers and celebrity trainer (clients have included Kevin Love, Kendall Jenner and Kate Beckinsale)*

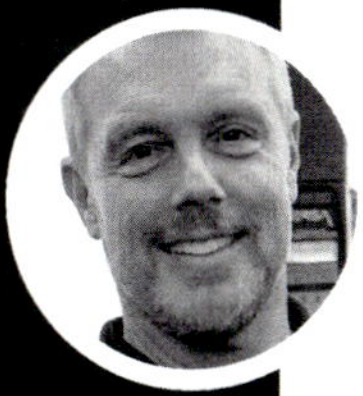

"Whenever you find yourself hitting the wall, don't accept it. Instead, take a few minutes to consider what's slowing you down. Ask yourself: Could it be fatigue? Dehydration? Monotony? Am I getting sick? All of the above! Sometimes, all it takes is a two-minute break to figure out what you need to address to break through that wall. If it's happening on a regular basis, try changing up the time of day you're working out."

8 Moves for a Strong Core

Building muscle improves your metabolism, bolsters the bones and helps prevent injury. In this excerpt from Lifted, trainer Holly Rilinger shares an abs routine

> ***By Holly Rilinger with Myatt Murphy***

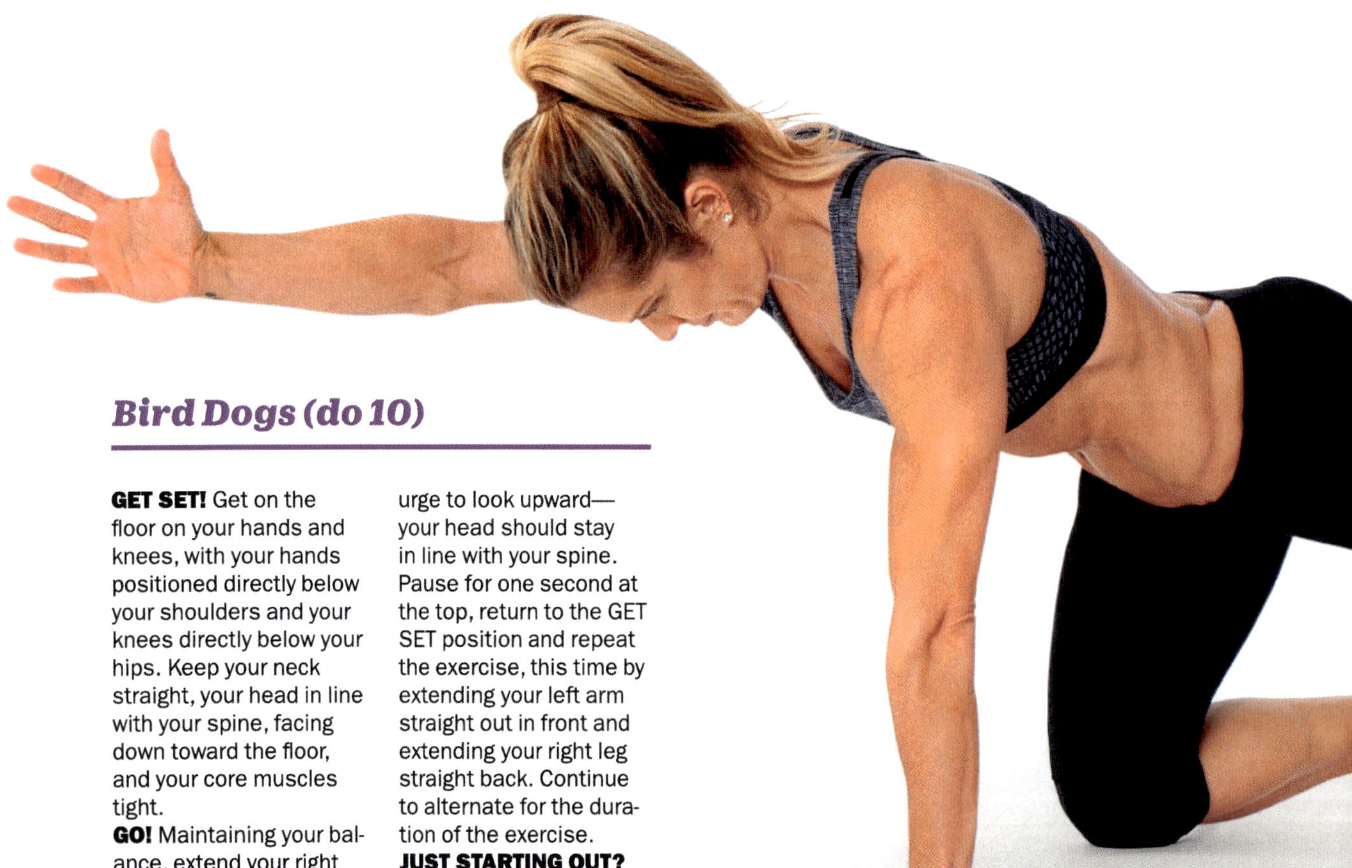

Bird Dogs (do 10)

GET SET! Get on the floor on your hands and knees, with your hands positioned directly below your shoulders and your knees directly below your hips. Keep your neck straight, your head in line with your spine, facing down toward the floor, and your core muscles tight.

GO! Maintaining your balance, extend your right arm straight out in front of you as you simultaneously extend your left leg straight back. Resist the urge to look upward—your head should stay in line with your spine. Pause for one second at the top, return to the GET SET position and repeat the exercise, this time by extending your left arm straight out in front and extending your right leg straight back. Continue to alternate for the duration of the exercise.

JUST STARTING OUT? Instead of extending one arm and one leg simultaneously, try doing one at a time.

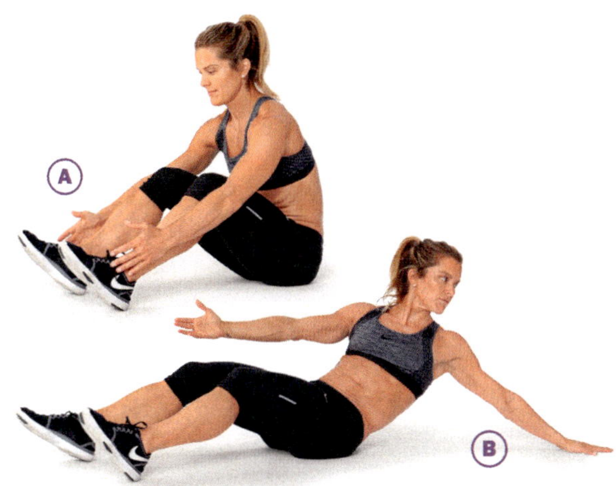

Reach Backs

GET SET! Begin by sitting on the floor with your legs bent in front of you, your toes raised and heels on the floor. Straighten arms in front of you, aiming your fingers toward your feet.
GO! With your core muscles braced for stability, keep your right arm pointing forward as you lean back and reach behind yourself as far as possible with your left hand. Try to stay focused on staying balanced on your butt as you go. Touch the floor with your left hand, then bring yourself back to the GET SET position. Repeat the exercise again, only this time keep your left arm pointed forward as you reach back with your right hand.
JUST STARTING OUT? If you're having a hard time balancing, try bending your legs more so your feet remain flat on the floor.

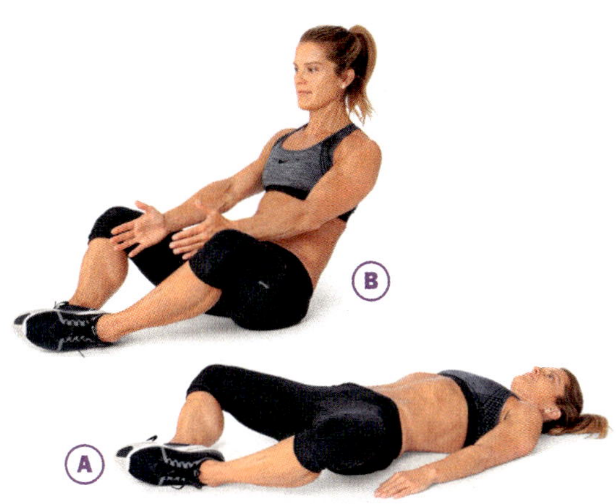

10 Goddess Sit-Ups

GET SET! Lie flat on your back with arms straight down at your sides, palms down. Place the soles of your feet together so your knees point out to the sides—this helps release your psoas, the deep muscles that connect your spine to your legs.
GO! Keeping soles of feet together, contract core muscles, then slowly curl your head, shoulders and back off the floor as you extend your arms forward toward your feet. Stop when your back is at about a 45-degree angle from the floor; lower yourself down into the GET SET position.
JUST STARTING OUT? Perform a normal crunch. Start with knees bent, feet flat on floor, and hands lightly touching behind your ears. Crunch up by raising head and shoulders off floor; lower yourself back down.

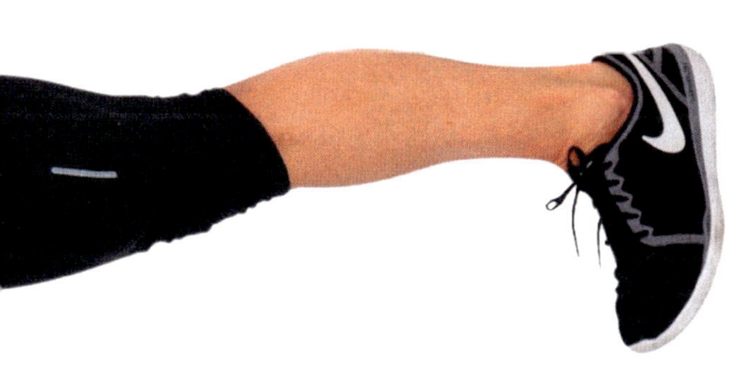

When doing this move, your head should stay in line with your spine.

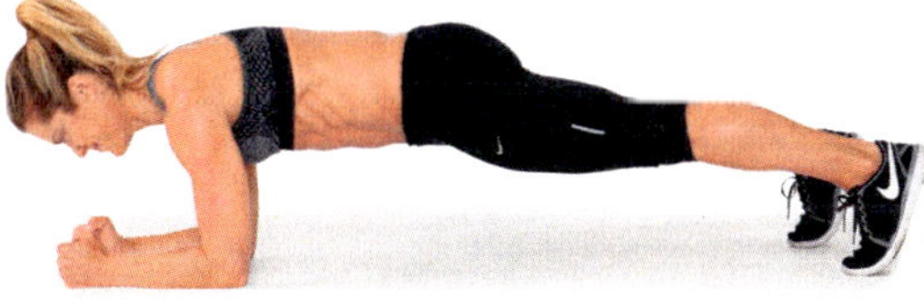

Planks (hold for 30 seconds)

GET SET! Get into position as if you were about to do a push-up, with your legs extended straight behind you, your weight resting on your toes and the balls of your feet. But instead of placing your hands on the floor, bend your arms and rest on your forearms. Your elbows should be directly below your shoulders, with your head facing down. Finally, pull in your stomach and tighten your core muscles.
GO! Actually, STAY! You'll hold position for 30 seconds. Your body should stay straight. If your hips drop, you'll place too much stress on your lower back. If your butt rises up too far, the move will be less effective.
JUST STARTING OUT? Try a modified plank by starting with your knees on the floor.

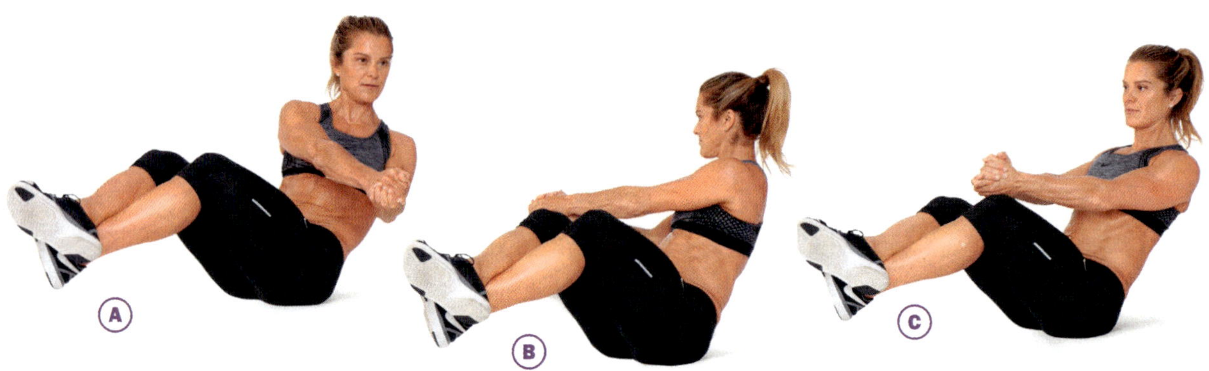

Russian Twists (30 seconds)

GET SET! Sit on the floor with your knees bent, your feet crossed and your heels raised off the floor. Straighten your arms out in front of you and clasp your hands, then slowly lean back until your torso is at a 45-degree angle. You should be balancing on just your butt.
GO! Keeping your arms straight and feet raised on the floor, slowly rotate to the right as far as you can without losing your balance. Return to the GET SET position, then repeat the move by slowly rotating to the left. Keep alternating back and forth throughout the exercise for the required amount of time.
JUST STARTING OUT? If you can't keep your balance, place your feet flat on the floor about shoulder width apart.

"The mind is the key to making lasting change to your body and spirit." —Rilinger

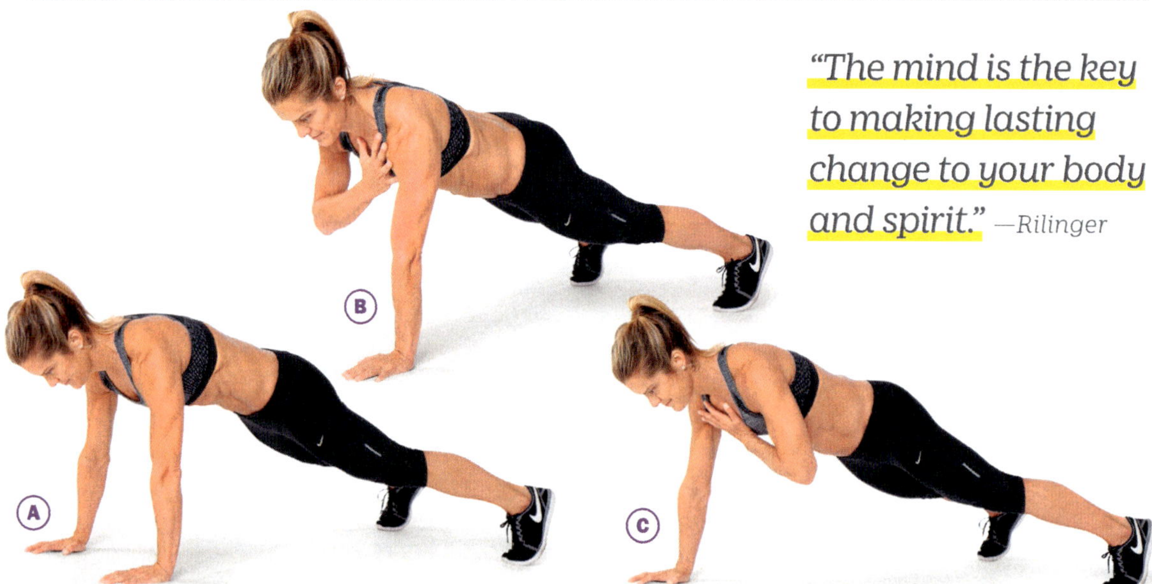

High Plank with Shoulder Taps (30 seconds)

GET SET! Get down on the floor in a push-up position, with your hands shoulder width apart and your legs extended behind you, feet also shoulder width apart.
GO! Maintaining your balance, shift your weight onto your right arm, then reach up with your left hand and touch your right shoulder. Place your hand back on the floor and repeat, this time shifting your weight onto your left arm and reaching up with your right hand to touch your left shoulder. Continue alternating back and forth for the duration of the exercise. As you go, don't allow your body to twist—your hips should remain square to the floor at all times.
JUST STARTING OUT? If you find it hard to maintain your balance, try the exercise with your knees on the ground. After you complete this routine, rest for 60 seconds, then start at the beginning and run through it again.

Fast Feet (30 seconds)

GET SET! Stand with your feet a few inches apart and up on the balls of your feet, heels raised. Your arms should be bent at 90 degrees, elbows tucked into your sides, with your palms facing down.

GO! Keeping your heels raised and arms up, step your feet up and down as quickly as you can—left foot, right foot. Don't raise your feet any higher than an inch from the floor—this move is about moving as quickly as possible, not lifting yourself any higher than you need to.

JUST STARTING OUT? Try the exercise at a slower pace.

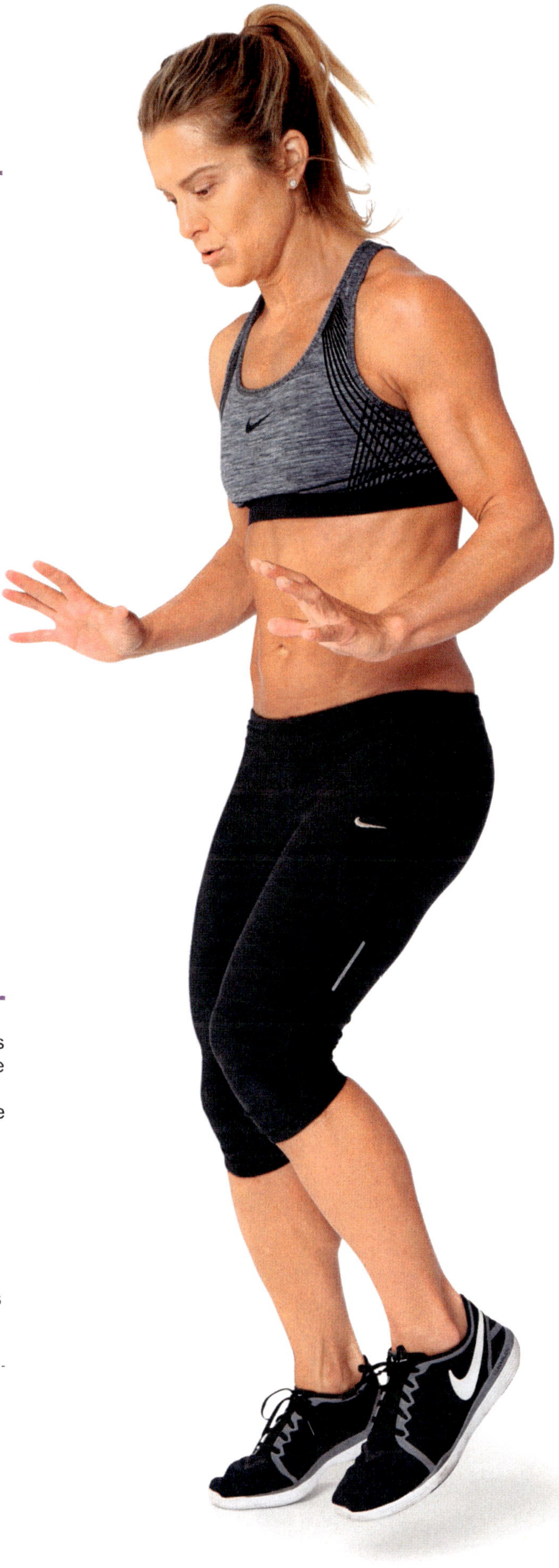

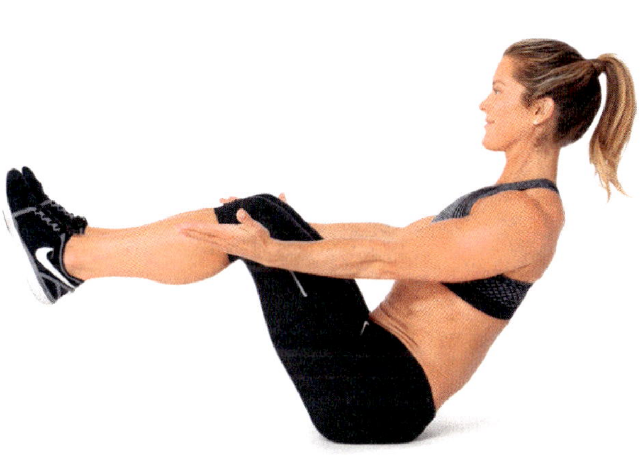

V-Ups (do 10)

GET SET! Lie flat on your back with your legs straight and your arms down by your sides.

GO! Keeping your back flat, simultaneously raise your knees and torso up so they are both at a 45-degree angle (your thighs and torso from the side should look like the letter V). As you rise, extend your arms forward, pointing your hands toward your feet. Reverse the motion by lowering yourself back down to the floor to return to the GET SET position.

JUST STARTING OUT? If you find it hard to balance or lack the core strength to come all the way up, just raise your legs and torso as high as you comfortably can.

The Tao of Being Round

Stressed about not having a six-pack? Abs, schmabs: there are far better reasons to work out

› By Dan Bova

I'VE BEEN BODY POSITIVE FOR MOST OF MY LIFE—positive that my body could be in way better shape.

And through the years, I've tried to do something about it. I've tried all kinds of diets. Low-carb, all carb, no meat, all meat. I even tried New England Patriots quarterback Tom Brady's diet . . . for exactly one day. I gave up not just because it was devoid of any possibility of joy (which it absolutely was) but also because it was really freaking complicated. Don't eat pineapples or tomatoes, but do eat swiss chard and avocado ice cream? Look, Tom, if I wanted to be confused, I'd go back to AP calculus and get a 1 on the final again.

I've also done all different kinds of workouts, hoping to get chiseled. Cardio kickboxing was fun until I took a punch (read: a light tap) to the jaw and had to excuse myself to go cry in the hallway. I've signed up for both stupidly expensive and weirdly cheap gym memberships (side note: is Planet Fitness collecting organs from us when we're not looking? How can it only be $10 a month? Nothing is $10 a month!). I've even—gasp!—walked to the store instead of driving to it in order to hit that daily goal of 10,000 steps that we have all been promised is the key to cardio health and possibly even world peace.

I've applied myself, and sure, after a few months I'll start to feel a little better. Hey, what's this odd en-

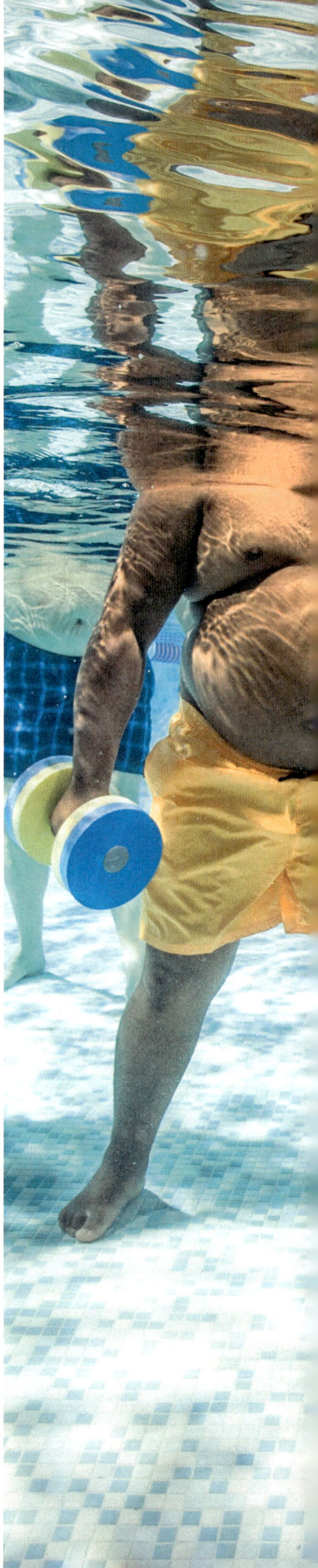

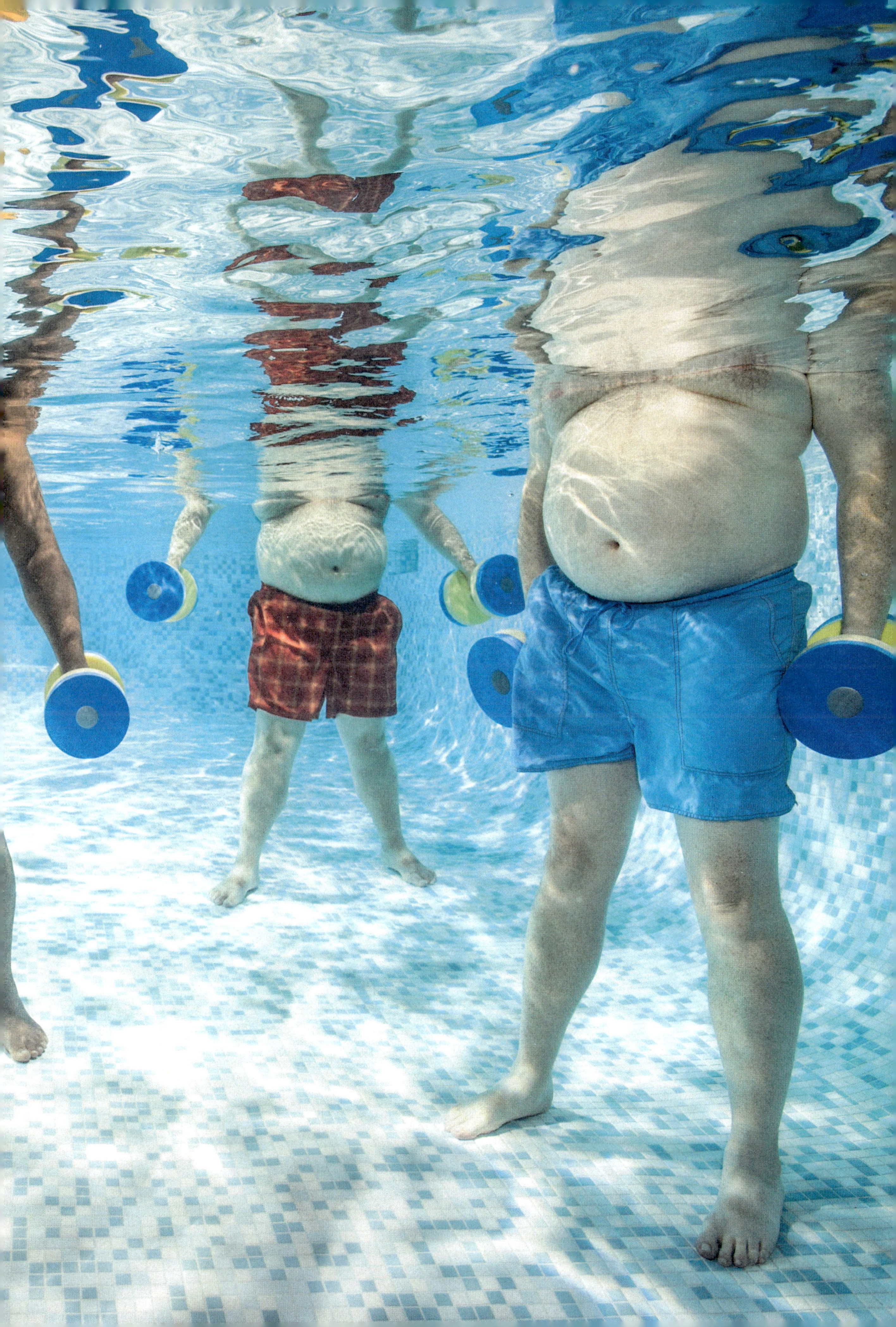

ergetic feeling I have? This is going great! But then I'll catch a glimpse of my midsection in the bathroom mirror and think, "C'mon, that's all you got for me?"

See, the thing is, I've always had something of a gut. It sticks to me like a wiggly, jiggly shadow whether I'm working out six days a week or not. Is that discouraging? Short answer: yes. Longer answer: holy crap yes! It seems like no matter what I do, my abs behave like a groundhog that saw its shadow and fled back into its burrow under my belly button. I'm 45 years old—will I go through life never having a six-pack?

Turns out, probably! So says Wayne L. Westcott, a professor of exercise science at Quincy College and co-author of *Strength Training Past 50*. "Most of us are genetically endowed with an average number of muscle cells and fat cells. But some people are born with a smaller-than-average number of muscle cells, and some people are born with more-than-average fat cells," he explains. "So they have to try to work through a thicker layer of fat to have their muscles—particularly the abs for men—pop through."

Westcott gave me a quick idiot-proof "Am I genetically blessed?" test that you can try too. Flex your biceps, and keep your forearm at a right angle. The average person can fit two index fingers between their biceps bulge and the crook of their elbow. But a *Men's Health* cover model? He can barely fit one. "They were born with a longer than average muscle belly, which is the sum of all the muscle fibers in any given muscle. And so they have greater potential to build bigger muscles."

In one study conducted by Claude Bouchard of Pennington Biomedical Research Center in Baton Rouge, La., a group of inactive men and women were put on an identical 20-week workout program and monitored to make sure they actually did it. And they did. At the end of the program, participants were measured for increases in endurance and ability to exercise at high-intensity levels, as well as changes in body fat and increases in muscle fiber. The result? Some improved a lot, and some didn't improve at all. And they all did the same thing!

But wait, it gets better. Not only do results vary from person to person, they can vary from muscle group to muscle group on the same person. Westcott tells the tale of legendary bodybuilder Boyer Coe, who competed in the '60s, '70s, '80s and '90s: "Interviewers would ask him, 'You have the best biceps in the world. What exercise do you do?' And he'd say, 'Doesn't matter—no matter what I do, it all works.' But they noticed he didn't have that six-pack, and they asked him, 'Don't you exercise your abs?' And he said, 'Yes, but it doesn't matter—whatever I do, it doesn't work!' And this was Mr. Universe! He was one of the best in the world, and even he couldn't overcome what genetics gave him."

While that all might sound discouraging, it is actually something of a relief. Genetics is to blame for my unsculpted shape. Woohoo! If my DNA hates sit-ups as much as I do, there's no need to exercise, right?

"Some people are born with a smaller-than-average number of muscle cells; some are born with more-than-average fat cells."

Wrong, Westcott is quick to answer. He and other experts are big proponents of strength training for the genetically blessed and messed alike. "There are a lot of good reasons to be doing strength training, and No. 1 is that people lose about six pounds of muscle per decade—even runners lose it if they don't strength train," Westcott says.

And a lack of muscle can result in more than just getting sand kicked in your face by buff beach bullies. Sarcopenia, the loss of muscle that comes with aging, brings with it a loss of bone, which can lead to osteoporosis (brittle bones). "That's what leads to broken bones and even death with some falls as people get older," Westcott notes.

Staving off bone loss is just one of the things pumping iron does. "Your muscles are the largest storehouse of sugar in the form of glycogen, so people who strength train have a much lower risk of Type 2 diabetes," Westcott says. Strength training also reduces your odds of developing high blood pressure, a risk factor for heart attacks and strokes.

OK, so I might not get killer arms from working out, but I also might eliminate getting a killer disease. Got it. So what now? Do I need to sign up for one of those crazy CrossFit classes where you hit big truck tires with sledgehammers for three hours? Just

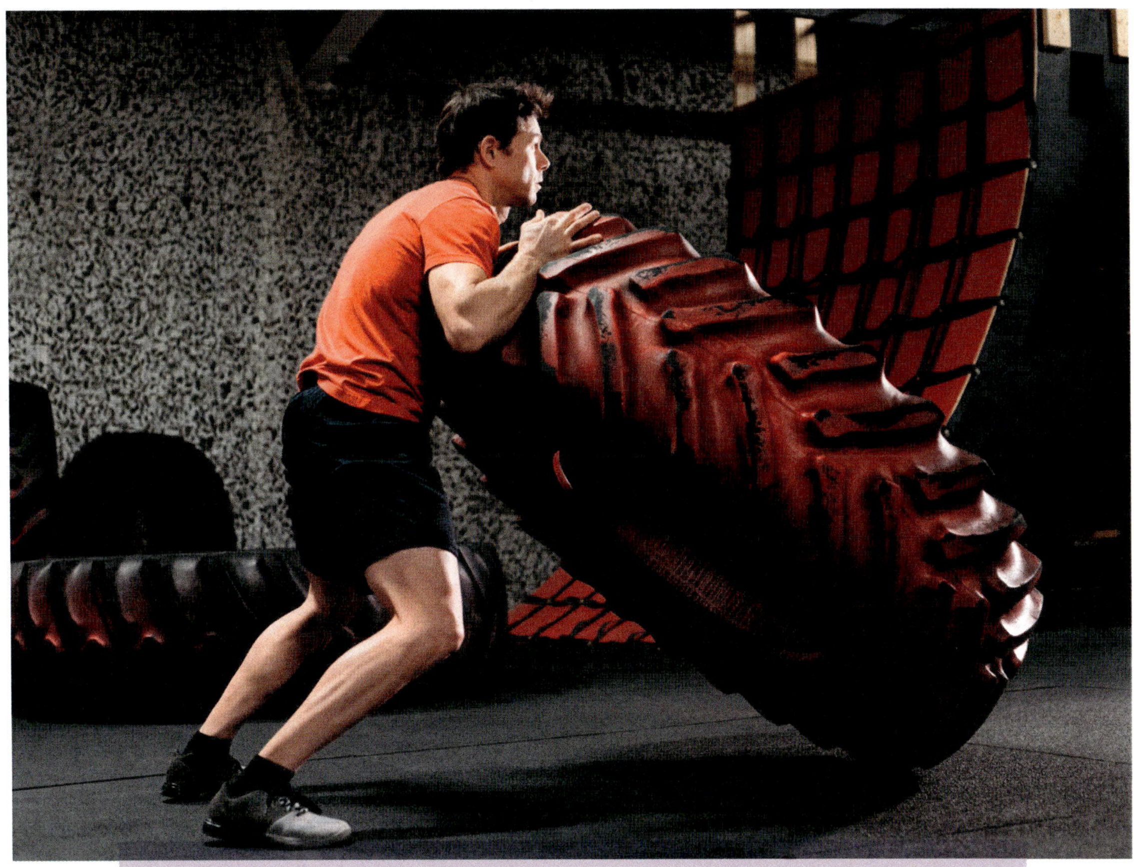

Good news: you don't have to endure extreme workouts to build significant muscle tone and improve your overall cardiovascular fitness.

the opposite, says Westcott. "Your body doesn't like major change—it wants homeostasis, to stay stable," he explains. "If you haven't been exercising, you need to start slow and gradually build up."

Results take time, adds Christi Pappas, a personal trainer in Commack, N.Y., who became a pro bodybuilder at the age of 46. "It is a marathon, not a sprint."

While you're patiently awaiting the day that your body is totally shredded, you can take comfort in this fact: you are building more muscle mass, which helps to shred calories. Even at rest, muscle tissue burns more calories than fat tissue. Not enough to throw in an extra Big Mac for dessert with no repercussions, but hell, I'll take any bonus burn I can get.

I asked Pappas for some exercise tips for people like me. Pappas gave me a dumbed-down weightlifting program. She refers to it as the push-and-pull plan. One day you do five exercises that all involve pushing: bench press, shoulder press, squats, triceps kickbacks, lunges—three sets of 20 repetitions with low weight. Then, in the next workout, you do all pulling moves: biceps curls, lat pull-downs, leg curls, stiff leg deadlifts, upright rows. Do this three or four days a week, mixing in 30 minutes of any kind of cardio you actually enjoy (or don't completely dread).

Since speaking to these exercise experts, I've re-started on my fitness journey with a whole new (more realistic) set of goals. Move over, six-pack; my new goal is to not have my knees sound like the floorboards of a haunted house whenever I stand up. And to not feel like I'm on the verge of a heart attack when I get to the top of the subway-station stairs. And guess what? Already nailed it! You hear that, gut? You and me are going places! □

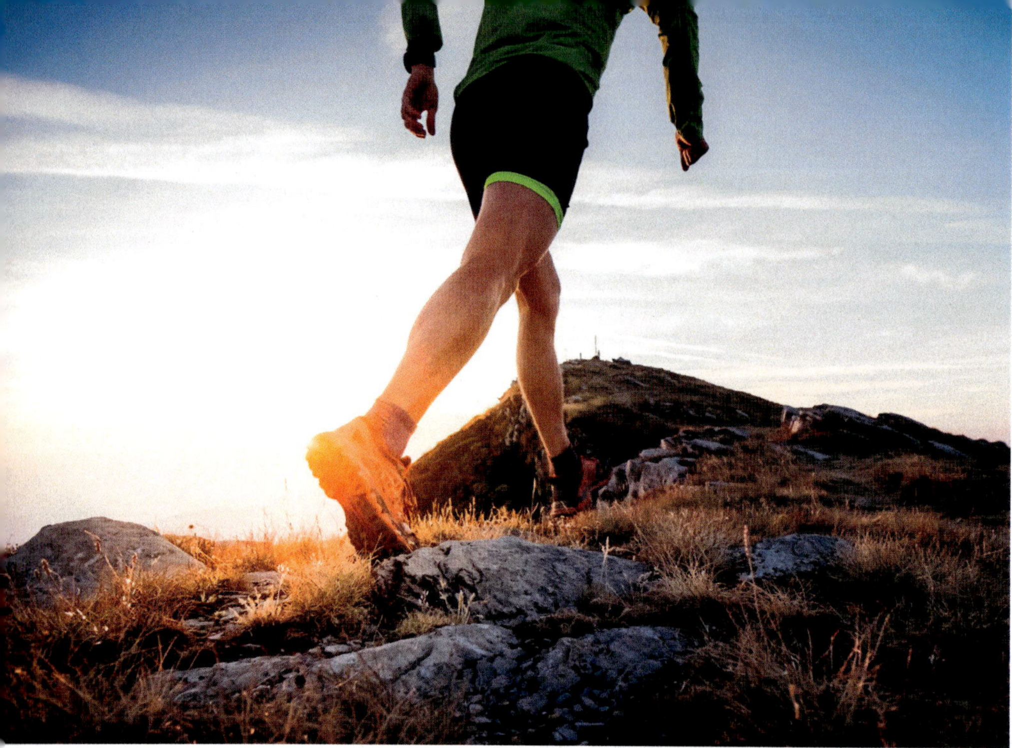

WHY NOT WALK?

It's the quick-stepping secret to dropping weight and staying fit for life BY JENNY EVERETT

When you want to shed weight, walking might not even come to mind. But it should.

"Fast-paced walking, when combined with healthy eating, is hugely effective for weight loss," says Art Weltman, director of exercise physiology at the University of Virginia. And those simple steps can have a big impact on your overall health, cutting your risk of everything from heart disease to depression. If your daily strolls haven't made you skinny so far, your speed may be the problem. Many of us stride more like a window-shopper than a power walker. The goal, thankfully, isn't crazy race-walker style; you just need to move at a challenging pace.

In studies, Weltman has found that women who do three short (about 30-minute) high-intensity walks plus two moderately paced recovery walks a week lose up to six times as much abdominal fat as participants who simply stroll five days a week. (This despite the fact that both groups burn the same number of calories.)

The power walkers also drop about four times as much total body fat. "There is a strong relationship between intensity of exercise and fat-burning hormones," says Weltman. "So if you're exercising at a pace considered to be hard, you're likely to release more of these hormones." The best part: when women walk, deep abdominal fat is the first to go.

Another happy truth: power walking is easier on the joints than running. "During walking, one of your feet is always in contact with the ground," says Weltman, "but during running, there's a float stage where your whole body is lifted in the air. Then you come back down and subject your body to the impact."

Dial In Your Speed

To make sure your pace is on point, use these guidelines from exercise physiologist Tom Holland, author of *Beat the Gym*. For maximum fat burn, aim for 30 minutes at power-walk intensity three days a week. You can complete it all at once or break it into spurts with recovery strides (stroll or brisk walk) in between.

> **Stroll:** Think window-shopping pace, or an intensity of 4 on a scale of 1 to 10. It burns about 238 calories an hour.

> **Brisk walk:** This means an effort of 5 or 6 on a scale of 1 to 10. It burns up to 340 calories an hour. While you can chat, you need to catch your breath every few sentences.

> **Power walk:** You're torching off about 564 calories an hour. Moving at this clip, using your arms to propel yourself forward, your effort should be 7 or 8 on a scale of 1 to 10. Talking is possible only in spurts of a few words, but . . . you'd . . . rather . . . focus . . . on . . . breathing.

Boost Your Benefit

> **Add hills.** When you hit the hills on a treadmill or in your neighborhood, you increase your calorie burn by nearly 20%, and that's just on a 1-degree to 5-degree incline.

> **Go off-road.** Head out for a light but brisk hike, and you'll torch approximately 430 calories in just an hour. Credit the uneven terrain, which forces you to work harder.

> **Swing your arms.** With your elbows bent at 90 degrees and hands in loose fists, move your arms in an arc, keeping elbows tight to your body. This helps drive you forward, builds upper-body strength and can increase your burn.

> **Focus on longer strides.** Instead of taking more steps, "work on increasing your stride length," Weltman advises. "You'll cover more ground," and that means more fat fried. □

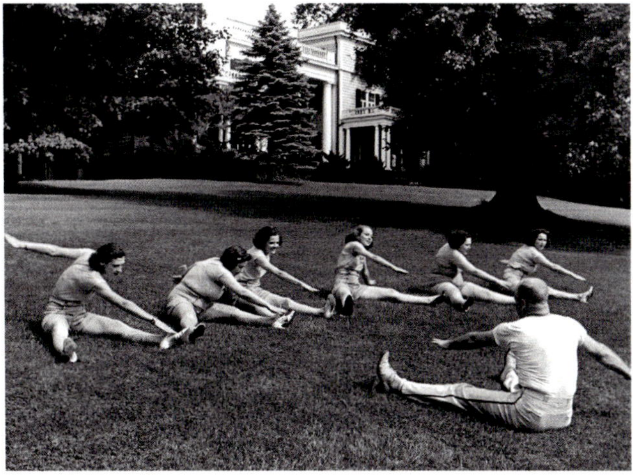

Women doing calisthenics at Rose Dor Farms, a weight-loss camp, in 1938

Credits

Front Cover
InnaKalyuzhina/iStock/Getty Images Plus; AngiePhotos/Getty Images

Back Cover
(clockwise from top left) pixelfit/Getty Images; Claudia Totir/Getty Images; Javier Snchez Mingorance/EyeEm/Getty Images; malerapaso/iStock/Getty Images Plus

Title Page
1 Dirima/Shutterstock

Contents
2–3 Rita Maas/Getty Images

Introduction
4 Rita Maas/Getty Images

Chapter 1: The New Think
6–7 Illustration by Libby Vander Ploeg **8–9** Alba Vitta/Addictive Creative/Offset **11** Phillip Harrington/Alamy **12** Vivian Zink/NBC/NBCU Photo Bank via Getty Images **15** Joshua Bright/The New York Times/Redux **17** Claudia Totir/Getty Images **19** Influx Productions/Getty Images **21** (chronological) James Keyser/The LIFE Images Collection/Getty Images; Andy Crawford/Getty Images; Ted Morrison/Getty Images; Evan Agostini/Getty Images; James Macari/Sports Illustrated **22–23** Chris Turner/Getty Images **25** Hugh Whitaker/Getty Images **26–27** The Good Brigade/Offset **28** zerocreatives/Westends61/Offset **30–31** jacoblund/Getty Images **33** ChristinLola/Getty Images **35** Shubhangi Ganeshrao Kene/Getty Images

Chapter 2: Clean Living
36–37 Illustration by Libby Vander Ploeg **38–39** RubberBall/Alamy **40** Juzant/Getty Images **42–43** DrGrounds/Getty Images **45** Peter Dazeley/Getty Images **46–51** Lucas Zarebinski for TIME (14) **52–53** (clockwise from top left) fongbeerredhot/Shutterstock; WAYHOME studio/Shutterstock; Tom Grill/Getty Images; LeoPatrizi/Getty Images **56–57** Rawpixel.com/Shutterstock **58** Silvia Otte/Getty Images **60** Anna Williams/Offset **62–63** Corey Rich/Aurora Photos/Alamy **65** UpperCut Images/Getty Images **66–67** Ryan Pfluger/AUGUST **68–69** Kathleen Multpeter (4) **70–71** Boris Jovanovic/Stocksy/Adobe Stock **73** santypan/Getty Images

Chapter 3: Power of Exercise
74–75 Illustration by Libby Vander Ploeg **76–77** Hero Images/Getty Images **78** Maridav/Getty Images **80–81** Taylor Jewell/Invision/AP/Shutterstock **81** (from top) Miller Mobley/AUGUST; Ilya S. Savenok/Getty Images for Lilly; Dimitrios Kambouris/Getty Images for Tiffany & Co.; Courtesy Melissa Alcantara **82** (from top) Tim P. Whitby/Getty Images for P.volve LLC; Magdalena Wosinska/The New York Times/Redux; Per Bernal **83** (from top) Maarten de Boer/Contour by Getty Images; Dave Kotinsky/Getty Images for FitBit **84** (from top) Art Streiber/NBC/NBCU Photo Bank via Getty Images; Courtesy Sebastien Lagree **85** (from top) Paras Griffin/WireImage/Getty Images; Chris Bull/Alamy; Jason Miller/Getty Images; Nicole Weingart/E! Entertainment/NBCU Photo Bank via Getty Images **86–89** Photographs by Matt Doyle (14) **90–91** Zena Holloway/Getty Images **93** Wavebreak Media/Offset **94** Simona Pilolla/Westend61/Offset

Masthead
95 Alfred Eisenstaedt/The LIFE Picture Collection/Getty Images

Shaping Up
96 (clockwise from top left) RLT_Images/Getty Images; bortonia/Getty Images; lumpynoodles/Getty Images (2); Vijay kumar/Getty Images

Published by Time Books, an imprint of Time Inc. Books, a division of Meredith Corporation.
225 Liberty Street · New York, NY 10281

Shaping Up: By the Numbers

9%

of American adults eat the recommended 2–3 cups of vegetables each day[9]

LESS THAN 5%

of adults get half an hour of physical activity every day[8]

100 GRAMS

Amount of protein the average American now eats daily—about twice as much as we need. Many people think they need to eat more protein to be healthier[7]

49%

Portion of American adults who are trying to lose weight[1]

19.5 teaspoons

Amount of added sugar the average American eats in one day[6]

10,000+

People listed in the National Weight Control Registry, which tracks people who have lost a significant amount of weight and kept it off for at least one year[5]

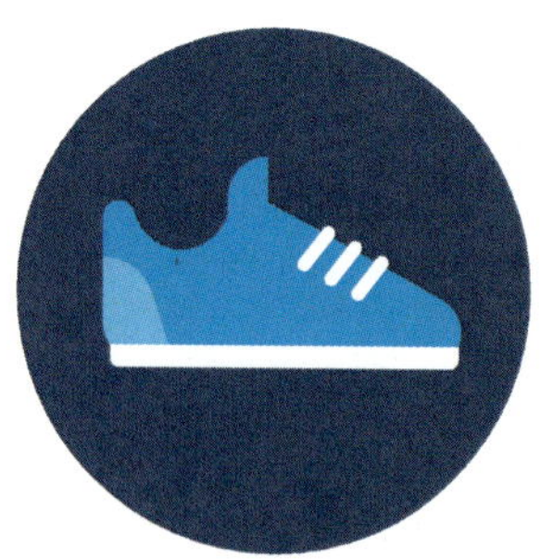

$900

Monthly fee at one high-end by-application-only gym in New York City[2]

$10

Monthly cost at a popular national gym chain[3]

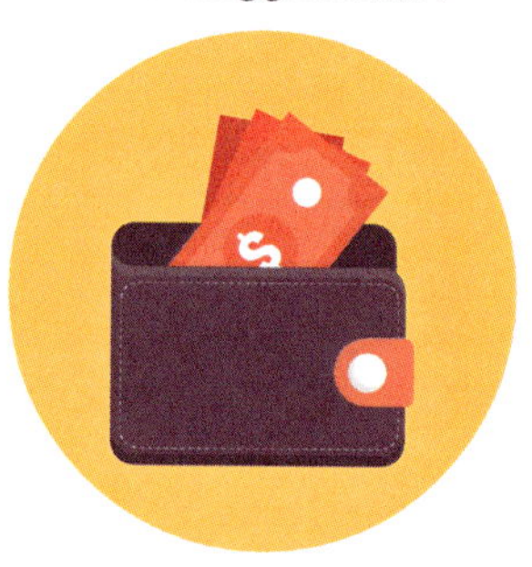

$9 BILLION

Value of the U.S. yogurt market[4]

SOURCES: (1) Centers for Disease Control and Prevention's National Center for Health Statistics (2) Forbes (3) Planet Fitness (4) Market-research firm Packaged Facts (5) National Weight Control Registry (6) University of California, San Francisco (7) The New York Times (8, 9) CDCSource: President's Council on Sports, Fitness and Nutrition

Made in the USA
Middletown, DE
05 March 2020